Dr. Ashley M. Berge, PhD
AM8 International
QLD, AUSTRALIA
+61 401 814 324
AM8@topicthread.com

THE SECRETS TO OPTIMAL
WELLBEING

a 12 week freestyle nutrition and functional
movement fitness guide

By

Dr. Ashley M. Berge, PhD

First published in 2016 by Dr. Ashley M. Berge, PhD
www.AM8International.com
Copyright © 2022 Ashley M. Berge
5th Edition
First published in 2016
ISBN: 978-0-9945694-5-5

DEDICATION

To all the specialists that endeavoured to help me regain my health yet were unable to provide me with answers, this is for you. May this Guide be used as a road map for all young adults on their journey to regaining their health.

To Faye, for always taking time to listen; for always taking time to understand; and for never giving up on me and my ailing health. I will always be indebted to the warmth and kindness you continue to show me.

And to You. Here's to happiness.

If you want to be happy, set a goal that commands your thoughts, liberates your energy, and inspires your hopes.

— Andrew Carnegie

FOREWORD

As a typical "sports" enthusiast I was the child that could always be found outside rather than inside. Training opposed to being "out" and about was the norm. From my early teenage years, I was consumed by my sport of choice, tennis, which dictated my schedule in the years to come. Ask those who know or knew me and they will argue how this "schedule" set the foundations for my past, present and future pursuits. This in itself led to *how I came to be*.

At 18, I became a Personal Trainer / Sports & Strength Conditioning Coach. I was also a full-time athlete, training for 8 hours a day.

At 19, I was a sponsored Elite Athlete. I also commenced University and maintained my full-time training.

At 20, I became a Level 1 Coach, then went on to become one of Australia's youngest ever Level 2 Coaches permitted to go back-to-back.

Just before I turned 21, I received a scholarship to play and train at one of America's leading Academies, in Texas.

At 21, I was coaching some of America's top national players as a direct result of succumbing to *another* injury whilst also playing and training – when healthy. That same year I received a full-scholarship to a National Collegiate Athletics Association (NCAA) DII private University that marked against the Harvard Grading Scale.

At 22, I spent part of the summer touring through Europe with American national players. At this time, I had also started my Undergraduate degree and had received a Grade Point Average (GPA) of a 4.0 (the highest attainable) in both first and second semesters. This came with multiple Dean's awards.

At 23, I spent part of the summer, again, touring through Europe with American national players. Due to injury, I had to fly back to Australia and leave my scholarship behind. I spent the majority of the year on crutches unable to walk. This was the year I completed my Undergraduate degree and started to run. This was also the year I had to choose between playing and coaching—I chose coaching.

At 24, I commenced my Masters. I spent the summer, once again, touring through Europe with American national players. On return I was asked to be the Director of a tennis program and accepted, being one of the youngest coaches, nationally, to take on such a position. After running for less than a year I managed to clock up 50 km days (not weeks). Just before I turned 25, I managed my biggest week yet: 180 km's in total.

At 25, I registered my business with my Dad and opted not to travel but to keep on top of my Masters (after receiving a GPA of 7.0: the highest attainable in Australia). Shortly after, my Dad passed away—just shy of my graduation; four months later, my Grandpa passed away.

At 26, I competed in my first Ultra race (100 km) but had a DNF (Did Not Finish) due to an ongoing hamstring injury. In the same year, I became recognised as a Level 3 Coach (the highest attainable globally). Soon after, I commenced my PhD – I still had questions to answer that my studies until then were unable to address.

At 27, my PhD was under full-swing and I was on track to complete my PhD in the minimum time frame. The same year I was able to sponsor my first athlete.

A fortnight after turning 28, I became unwell. Ultimately, I couldn't run, walk, read, write, do simple tasks, let alone finish the home-stretch of my PhD without near-collapsing. Without going into detail, somehow I did manage to finish my PhD and in the minimum time frame; with only four months leave taken.

But this left me awestruck – quite literally. Sometimes it takes losing something to truly realise and appreciate its worth. Never in my wildest dreams did I ever think that it would be my health. Nor did I think it would ever be "hard" let alone unheard of to those I was seeking help from (specialists and practicians from every avenue) to be unable to help me. And thus my "new" research journey began.

At 29, I had PhD corrections to look after, although the entire year was all about getting my health back. Not only was I finalising my PhD (corrections) I was also religiously looking left, right and centre into any avenue that could tell me what was happening to my body, and what had caused it.

These answers eventually came. The facial and cranial pain I was experiencing was later identified as an impinged cranial nerve inflicted by a dental procedure, causing severe nerve trauma. In attempt to alleviate this I had surgery that could have left me far-worse off.

Today, half way through my 30th year and a little over a year since the surgery at the time of publication, I am incredibly fortunate to still be here. Those who were there for me find it hard to fathom that I am still alive – something I still find hard to swallow. Risks can, and do pay off.

The surgery was not the answer to everything. Due to the longevity of the trauma additional complications arose. These were later identified as severe gut disruptions. This was highlighted when I competed in my first Ultra since becoming unwell, and although mere months prior to the surgery, I finished all 80 km's of it whilst my gut was inflamed and my head experiencing what can only be described as a 24/7 ongoing migraine. This later was aligned with a constant chronic cough I had developed, sporadic rashes over my body, breathing disruptions and an increase in body temperature – and other minor ailments.

My new research journey had identified causations which were mind boggling. So I made a decision: to fight this – if no professional could help me, I was going to help myself by finding an answer and a solution. No longer did I want to be weak and left at the demise of my ailing health – I wanted to regain my health, I wanted to take control of my life again: I decided to choose *happiness*.

With my PhD journey coming to an end, this "other" journey had just begun. And I found my answer. Little did I know that "all" of these health-related symptoms that peaked from severe intensities through to daily plateaus, were in fact related to my gut and the trauma it in itself endured at the hands of overprescribed medications – yet a direct cause-effect from the incorrect treatment of my initial health demise – cranial nerve impingement. With the surgery been and gone, there lied my solution: gut restoration.

A year has passed since my gut health began to restore itself, a continuing process, but equally my choice – to choose happiness. This Guide has been formed for you to choose too – I can confidently say that the "keys" identified in my gut rehabilitation and restoration process, discussed herein, have contributed immensely to my personal health and wellbeing.

Although trauma from the surgery remains, it has improved. The consequences of my health deteriorating, primarily gut disruptions inflicted by foreign prescribed medicines, have improved immensely. And by making the decision to choose happiness – this in itself has been life reaffirming. Not only do I feel healthier in myself through adopting this Guide, to come, but it has put me on the road to recovering completely, in time, and discovering so much more.

Gut trauma can be managed and near-rectified in time. This time is a process and "my" time has come in leaps and bounds. So much so, as an Ultra runner this Guide allows me to not only clock up 100km's plus on a weekly basis, but by following it 80% of the time, whereby balance is key, I have more energy and feel even healthier than before. Of course, the trauma still remains from the surgery, but this Guide allows it to be managed without the complications associated with the gut ailments and intense disruptions.

Over time, through following this Guide I became aware of "triggers" – foods that I reacted to and caused my gut to "run havoc" whilst other foods that allowed my gut to quite simply "be" and leave me at ease. Thus, by following this Guide 80% of the time now, compared to 100% of the time a year ago, these triggers occur based on the simple rule of moderation – yes, you can *have your cake and eat it too* – because, happiness!

The two components that form this Guide are the freestyle nutrition and functional movement fitness. The nutrition is centred on giving you the "tools" to create – to take control over your nutrition and design it the way *you* choose – freestyling! The functional movement fitness is drawn from my background as a Sports Scientist, Strength and Conditioning Coach, and one of the world's *leading* coaching professionals on how to "move" and "perform" – exercises from home feature, with ease, that use more than one muscle-group at a time, employing functional movement principles. The outcome is a reduced risk of injury, a program that is time efficient, and movements that reflect and are applied in our day to day lives – thus applicability to perform.

Herein is a Guide for you to use as your own personal template towards your *fitter* and *healthier* lifestyle. This is a lifestyle change. I was *forced* to alter my lifestyle at the detriment of a health complication. But you have a **choice**. The best medicine for *optimal wellbeing* is *fitness* – physical activities that "switch" your gut into a cleansing mode whilst also releasing endorphins to give you those "feel good" vibes likened to a great night out! And your *nutrition* – using food as "fuel" – your energy source for leading a happier and healthier lifestyle!

To follow is an outline of how this Guide works in conjunction with you – your *optimal wellbeing*. Your Guide caters for your *fitness* and *nutrition*, giving you the reins to control your ultimate *wellbeing* and its longevity. And remember: choose happiness.

I truly hope that you take away, from this book, as much as I have learned when compiling it over the past year – through the countless questions and naïve specialists encountered that lead to in-depth research on how to not only fuel myself, but to ensure our guts are well cared for in a balanced light – we all want our cake too! Herein I share the answers to those secrets I wanted to know so dearly to regain my optimal wellbeing. To all the young adults especially, here's to putting into action the building blocks for the lifestyle you've always desired – health is wealth!

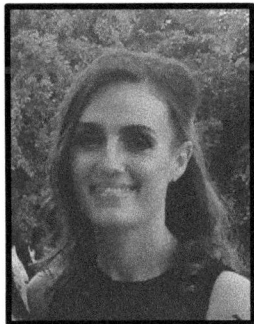

Dr. Ashley M. Berge is currently the world's leading expert on the forehand groundstroke, effective December 2016. She is also inside the top 1% of coaches globally for her tennis-specific knowledge and expertise, and specifically for her age and gender.

CONTENTS

THE SECRETS TO OPTIMAL
WELLBEING

a 12 week freestyle nutrition and functional
movement fitness guide

By

Dr. Ashley M. Berge, PhD

PART 1

THE ROAD MAP

Outline

Two of the most contested topics that "anyone" and "everyone" has an opinion on are *fitness* and *nutrition*. A result of countless health epidemics that have come to light over the years, the most sacred "health" concern is taking back control over your body – picking up the reins to control what you have the capacity to: your happiness.

Enter "fitness" or "nutrition" into a search engine and the results will be endless. If you're like me you will find copious resources, yet conflicting opinions on *both* fitness and nutrition foundations, implications and personalised applicability. It is tiresome. It is mindboggling at the best of times. And new "fads" appear to pop up on a daily basis.

But what about you? What about *you* taking responsibility for your own *wellbeing* and taking back *control* that so many fitness and nutrition "fads" remove? How about you rewiring your mindset on fitness and nutrition by way of "freestyling" through your own recipes with the "keys" given to adopt a healthier and fitter version of you? And what about learning how to execute fitness orientated activities and exercises "functionally" by being shown functional movements – movements that have your body "move" how it was designed, in its natural state, ensuring the risk of injury is minimised. What's more, these movements draw on more than one muscle-group – thus ultimately minimising the time spent exercising.

Welcome to the premise of this Guide. It is all about giving you the "keys" for 12 Weeks and setting you up to "freestyle" your nutrition and teach you how to "move" – at home or wherever you desire without the need for ongoing memberships. This Guide is designed for you – for you to take the reins of your lifestyle and to keep the choice of happiness at the forefront, or rather your front pocket, always.

1.1 It's a Guide

The essence of *The Secrets to Optimal Wellbeing* is that first and foremost, it is a Guide. It is to be used to implement the "keys" necessary to achieve a healthy bodily response to both fitness *and* nutrition. It is key to recognise that these work in collaboration – your *optimal wellbeing* is a result of putting in place a fitness and nutrition lifestyle that works for you, an end result of choosing happiness.

The Guide has been designed for the young adult as a trajectory for taking the reins of their wellbeing. As with all lifestyle deviations, it is always a good idea to check with your local doctor that you're ready to undertake any form or level of fitness and their ultimate implications when implementing a new nutrition and/or fitness Guide.

The nutrition component of this Guide, featured in Part 2, has been formed on the basis of *simplicity* and *efficiency* – recipes can be prepared more often than not in a timely manner, they work *with you* towards your gut health, they provide the building blocks for you to personalise and create your *own* meals with weekend freedom – to apply your newfound knowledge, plus, you literally get to have your cake and eat it too!

The fitness component of this Guide, presented in Part 3, has been designed from a beginner basis. That is, for those starting from scratch, this is specifically for you. For those who have a reasonable level of fitness, this Guide is also applicable allowing *you* to work towards your own individual level of fitness. However, this Guide has not been designed for the athlete or heavily trained fitness enthusiast with the want to push themselves one step further – this Guide *gives you* the "tools" to be able to do so once you have mastered and accomplished the building blocks and set foundations of this fitness Guide.

1.2 Mix & Match

The power is yours. Part 4 is where the 12 Week Guide begins, whilst Parts 2 and 3 comprise of the "keys" to transition this Guide into taking the reins of your lifestyle, which is reaffirmed come Part 5, post 12 Week implementation. This is about you and giving *you* your freedom – to freestyle through the recipes provided in Part 2 and to take control of what you choose to "create" and "make" on the weekends, whilst also asserting trust in you. The same applies to your fitness and the functional movement parameters discussed in Part 3 – trust in yourself to apply, trust in yourself to commit, and trust in yourself to see it through, for *you*. That's right – trust; trust in your decisions and choices.

The Guide has intentionally given you the power to *choose* what you want to have for breakfast and *what* you fuel yourself with over the weekend. It is important to be mindful of this freedom and that you are *learning* the keys to achieve and maintain your *optimal wellbeing*. There is freedom to choose your "snacks" with recipes provided, yet tangibility to mix *and* match what snacks *you choose* to have and when. Freedom also comes in time – you choose when to *implement* your fitness Guide, you choose where, and you choose the times you put aside to *execute* it as designed.

This is about you and trusting in yourself to make the right decisions for *you*. There is no right or wrong answer, but there are better *choices* when it comes to you controlling your *optimal wellbeing*. The Guide is to be used as just that – a Guide to regaining control *and* awareness over your gut, its health, and ensuring you stay fit and active, contributing to your ultimate *wellbeing*.

1.3 Layout with Personal Power

Time is one of the leading causes for disruption. That is, disruption of our lifestyle and disruption for our *optimal wellbeing*. This Guide has taken time and given you back the *power* to personalise your nutrition and fitness on your terms – with minimal time, limiting the influence of this disruption.

Part 2 is where the nutrition component of the Guide is presented with raw, vegan, gluten-free, vegetarian and meat-based recipes *all* inclusive. A heavy emphasis has been placed on vegetarian recipes with simple underpinnings if you so choose to make them raw, vegan *or* meat-based, with all but a handful of recipes gluten-free and easily interchangeable.

In order to restore your gut and to become aware of *how* it responds to your nutrition choices, we need to cut back foods that are not as easily digested – this includes meat-based recipes. Thus, these are included throughout the 12 Week Plan, yet kept to a minimum. Recipes can easily be made raw by removing cooked ingredients – this will become more notable as the week's progress and you become more aware of how simple this becomes. As for vegan, the majority of recipes presented *are* in fact vegan with the exception for added condiments and flavours. These are easily customisable and interchangeable, which again you will become more aware of as the week's progress.

The best part? The majority of *all* recipes take less than 20 minutes to prepare. And for those of you like me that prefer a minimal-fuss clean that comes *after* the cooking, this too has been considered to ensure time is on your side and there's no kitchen storm to clear!

Now for the real power. Part 3 is where the fitness component of the Guide is presented – in discussion of "how" to perform specific exercises. This section acts as a reference point for the 12 Weeks ahead and beyond, specifically when it comes to "performing" at-home exercises with minimal fuss and minimal equipment. The equipment to be used has been chosen for the homeward bound young adult with "bits" and "pieces" primarily around the home that can be used and turned into a fitness tool.

The fitness component of the Guide is in your hands. You have the power to choose when *and* where. The Guide provides days *and* the duration of each activity – strength and aerobic, with the strength plan to be implemented 3-5 days per week, and the aerobic plan implemented 4-5 days per week. You *do* get days off, you *do* get to choose when, and you *do* get time to rest and recover throughout the week.

It is important to remember and note throughout your 12 Week Journey that at any time if you're unsure of "how" to perform, or if you're unsure of "how" to prepare any of your meals, to just ask! Social media is there for a reason and so is AM8International.com and its array of contact options. So please, if ever in doubt – ask away.

1.4 12 Weeks towards a Healthier and Fitter You

Heed this warning: you will have times of doubt. You will have times where your desires and temptations get the better of you. But, I am telling you now – it's okay! Over the next 12 Weeks you have options for your snacks which include the indulgence of cake, or *whatever* sweet treat you have been saving up to devour!

Remember, it's about a lifestyle change – giving you the power to choose and control your fitness *and* nutrition, once and for all, further discussed in Part 5, *post* journey. This means if some days you're a little more tired than others, you can switch your fitness times around by simply *ensuring* you hit and stick to your weekly commitment i.e. 3-5 times per week depending on the "week" you have progressed towards. It is also a reminder that your breakfasts and weekend meals are up to you – they're in your hands.

Over the weeks you will begin to learn "what" your body wants, "how" your body responds to different food sources, and also what works "best" for you – this is *all* about you and *not one person* will be the same. Some of you will favour "one" food source more than another, whilst others will be the complete opposite – and that's okay. The key here is to learn what your body wants – how your body reacts, and to begin to understand *The Secrets to Optimal Wellbeing*.

Closing thoughts

Remember: it is a Guide – and you're the director. This Guide has been designed for *you* with the intention of giving you the *tools*, showing you the *keys*, and setting you free – free to choose, free to create, and free to choose your own revamped lifestyle. The layout is now in your hands with the capacity to personalise the Guide – from mixing and matching to allocating the time you choose to put *towards a healthier and fitter you.*

The time has come for your 12 Weeks to begin. Let this 12 Weeks be a reminder of how powerful you are – you have the power to control your freedom. You have the power to control your happiness. And most of all, you have the power to control your lifestyle: *towards a healthier and fitter you.*

PART 2

FREESTYLE NUTRITION

Outline

Too often than not it is perceived that "making" what we choose to eat is not only time consuming, but as a result of all the "fads" it is often treaded with caution. Questions often asked include whether or not I am allowed to eat this? Will this make me fat? Will this make my tummy bigger? Am I allowed to have a bit more?

At the end of the day, what we are told is so confusing, so conflicting, that we become lost in the maze of diet *verse* nutrition rather than perceiving our *health* as just that – what make you feel healthy *and* happy? Yes, the two "ideologies" work hand in hand – healthy body, healthy mind, healthy being – contributing towards your *optimal wellbeing.*

Part 2 is set out in 5 segments: 2.1 comprises of meals that are distinctly raw, gluten-free and vegan – *all* in one. Come 2.2 you will find 80% of *all* meals and where you will find the "building blocks" of your meals. Section 2.2 plays hand-in-hand with section 2.1 providing vegetarian dishes that have only moderately been adapted from vegan and raw based recipes.

The majority of all recipes provided are gluten-free with the exception of section 2.3 where primarily muffin recipes are presented. To ensure recipes are gluten-free, this can easily be done simply by substituting standard flour to gluten-free flour – the *choice* is yours.

Come 2.4 you will find smoothie recipes that are suggested throughout your week as "snacks" (not meal replacements). This is to ensure you're not only getting a solid dose of vitamins and minerals, but to show you how simply and easy it can be to adopt a healthier and fitter lifestyle wherever your life may take you.

To end Part 2, you will find in 2.5 meat-based meals that primarily include chicken and fish in the recipes presented with the option to *always* substitute. This means that if you don't fancy chicken but would like beef, you can; the same applies if you'd prefer lamb rather than fish – yes, you can. The key is for you to choose what's best for you whilst also ensuring you are substituting an "apple for an apple" and not an "orange for a pear" – chicken and fish have been used to provide easy and tangible recipes that you can take the reins of and personalise by choice of protein.

Let your journey to freestyle nutrition begin!

2.1 Raw, Gluten-Free & Vegan

The recipes featured in 2.1 are all raw (optional), vegan *and* gluten-free. The condiments used in all recipes *are* vegan-friendly and as a result of recipes being raw – they're quick, easy, and *no cooking* is required (options provided). The objective of this section is to provide the foundations of vegan nutrition and to give you the freedom to *choose* whilst *learning* about the ingredients and condiments that work *for* you – it is your freedom to choose.

Featured Recipes:

Beetroot & Sprout Salad
Cabbage & Beetroot Salad
Cabbage & Olive Salad
Lentil & Bean Mixed Salad
Tofu Salad
Zucchini & Avocado Salad
Kale & Apple Salad
Kale & Beetroot Salad
Celery & Beetroot Salad
Carrot & Kale Salad

2.1.1 Beetroot & Sprout Salad

Ingredients:
Chia Seeds (few sprinkles)
Kale (1 stem)
Cabbage (1/2 cup)
Bean Sprouts (1/2 cup)
Carrots (1)
Beetroot (1/2 cup)
Olive Oil (drizzle)

Preparation time:
15 minutes

Serves:
1

Nutrition friendly:
Raw
Gluten-Free
Vegan
Vegetarian

Guide:
Slice kale finely.
Slice cabbage finely.
Chop carrots and beetroot into cubes.
Add bean sprouts and all other ingredients to salad bowl.
Add chia seeds and drizzle with olive oil.
Done!

Tag your salad on Topicthread to be added to our gallery!
https://am8international.com/health-gallery

2.1.2 Cabbage & Beetroot Salad

Ingredients:
Beetroot (1/2 cup)
Avocado (1/2)
Kale (1 stem)
Cabbage (1/2 cup)
Zucchini (1/4 cup)
Ginger (centimetre)
Garlic (1 clove)
Olive Oil

Preparation time:
20 minutes

Serves:
1

Nutrition friendly:
Raw
Gluten-Free
Vegan
Vegetarian

Guide:
Slice beetroot, avocado and zucchini (steamed, optional) into cubes.
Finely slice kale and cabbage followed by finely slicing the ginger and garlic.
Add all ingredients to salad bowl and drizzle with olive oil.
Done!

Tag your salad on Topicthread to be added to our gallery!

2.1.3 Cabbage & Olive Salad

Ingredients:
Chia Seeds (few sprinkles)
Cabbage (1 cup)
Carrot (1 cup)
Olives, Black (1/4 cup)
Tomato (1)
Garlic (1 clove)
Olive Oil

Preparation time:
15 minutes

Serves:
1

Nutrition friendly:
Raw
Gluten-Free
Vegan
Vegetarian

Guide:
Slice cabbage finely.
Chop tomato and carrot into cubes.
Slice olives finely along with garlic clove.
Add all ingredients to salad bowl and sprinkle with chia
seeds.
Stir through all ingredients and dress with olive oil.
Done!

Tag your salad on Topicthread to be added to our gallery!

2.1.4 Carrot & Kale Salad

Ingredients:
Kale (1 stem)
Beetroot (1/3 cup)
Capsicum (1/2)
Carrots (1)
Mayonnaise (vegan friendly)

Preparation time:
10 minutes

Serves:
1

Nutrition friendly:
Raw
Gluten-Free
Vegan
Vegetarian

Guide:
Pull a part kale into edible chunks.
Chop beetroot, capsicum and carrot into cubes.
Add all ingredients to salad bowl.
Stir through and dress with mayonnaise.
Done!

Tag your salad on Topicthread to be added to our gallery!

2.1.5 Celery & Beetroot Salad

Ingredients:
Sauerkraut (handful)
Celery (2 sticks)
Kidney Beans (1/2 cup)
Beetroot (1/2 cup)
Garlic (2 cloves)

Preparation time:
15 minutes

Serves:
1

Nutrition friendly:
Raw
Gluten-Free
Vegan
Vegetarian

Guide:
Rinse kidney beans and place into salad bowl.
Chop celery into fine pieces – add to bowl.
Slice beetroot (your choice of fresh or canned – if fresh
cook through until tender) into cubes – add to bowl.
Add sauerkraut to bowl after chopping into edible-length
pieces.
Add garlic (raw) to bowl.
Done!

Tag your salad on Topicthread to be added to our gallery!

2.1.6 Kale & Apple Salad

Ingredients:
Kale (2 stems/bunches)
Apple (1)
Orange (1)
Garlic (2 cloves)
Cabbage (1 cup)

Preparation time:
15 minutes

Serves:
1

Nutrition friendly:
Raw
Gluten-Free
Vegan
Vegetarian

Guide:
Rinse kale and chop into fine slices.
Chop cabbage finely.
Slice apple and orange into cubes.
Slice garlic finely.
Add all ingredients to salad bowl – toss through.
Done!

Tag your salad on Topicthread to be added to our gallery!

2.1.7 Kale & Beetroot Salad

Ingredients:
Kale (1 stem)
Capsicum (1/2)
Carrot (1)
Potato (2 small)
Mixed Beans (1/4 cup)
Beetroot (1/2 cup)
Broccoli (1/4 cup)
Mushrooms (1/4 cup)
Olive Oil (to serve)

Preparation time:
20 minutes

Serves:
1

Nutrition friendly:
Raw
Gluten-Free
Vegan
Vegetarian

Guide:
Chop potato into chunks – add to microwave safe dish and cook through (stove top option available). Once cooked, rinse with cold water. Let potatoes cool then chop into finer cubes.
Slice kale and mushrooms finely.
Chop capsicum, carrot and beetroot into cubes.
Chop broccoli into edible pieces.
Rinse beans and add to salad bowl along with all other ingredients – drizzle with olive oil.
Done!

Tag your salad on Topicthread to be added to our gallery!

2.1.8 Lentil & Bean Mixed Salad

Ingredients:
Lentils (1/3 cup)
Kale (1 stem)
Kidney Beans, Mixed (1/3 cup)
Beetroot (1/3 cup)
Pineapple (1/3 cup)
Tomato (1)
Mayonnaise (vegan friendly option)

Preparation time:
20 minutes

Serves:
1

Nutrition friendly:
Raw
Gluten-Free
Vegan
Vegetarian

Guide:
Drain and rinse lentils thoroughly – add to salad bowl.
Drain and rinse kidney beans thoroughly – add to salad bowl.
Slice kale finely.
Chop tomato and beetroot into cubes.
Slice pineapple into cubes – add all ingredients to salad bowl.
Stir through and add mayonnaise to dress.
Done!

Tag your salad on Topicthread to be added to our gallery!

2.1.9 Tofu Salad

Ingredients:

Tofu (100g, optional)
Tomato (1)
Mushrooms (1/2 cup)
Cabbage (1/2 cup)
Broccoli (1/2 cup)
Spiced Olives (20g)

Pickled Ginger (20g)
Chilli Flakes (few sprinkles)
Salt and Pepper (to season)

Preparation time:
20 minutes

Serves:
1

Nutrition friendly:
Raw
Gluten-Free
Vegan
Vegetarian

Guide:
Slice tofu (optional) into cubes and add to bowl.
Add salt and pepper to bowl along with chilli flakes to season tofu.
Slice mushrooms finely.
Chop tomato into cubes.
Slice cabbage and olives finely.
Chop broccoli into small pieces.
Add pickled ginger to bowl along with all other ingredients – stir through and add salt, pepper and chilli flakes to taste.
Done!

Tag your salad on Topicthread to be added to our gallery!

2.1.10 Zucchini & Avocado Salad

Ingredients:
Kale (1 stem)
Cabbage (1 cup)
Avocado (1/2)
Zucchini (1/3 cup)
Bean Sprouts (1/2 cup)
Olive Oil

Preparation time:
15 minutes

Serves:
1

Nutrition friendly:
Raw
Gluten-Free
Vegan
Vegetarian

Guide:
Slice kale and cabbage finely and add to salad bowl.
Chop avocado and zucchini (steamed, optional) into cubes.
Add bean sprouts, avocado and zucchini to salad bowl.
Stir through ingredients and dress with olive oil.
Done!

Tag your salad on Topicthread to be added to our gallery!

2.2 Vegetarian, Vegetable Salads & Stir-Fry's

The recipes presented in 2.2 are all vegetarian with a combination of stir-fry's and salads. All recipes can be easily made vegan (predominantly by substituting condiments) and can be made raw by *choice*. The recipes too are *primarily* gluten-free. To remove all gluten, simply substitute with your personal preference, for example, white bread to a gluten-free bread.

Featured Recipes:

Bean & Sweet Potato Salad
Broccoli & Olive Pasta
Cabbage & Beans
Cabbage & Mushroom Pasta Salad
Cabbage & Pickle Salad
Cabbage & Brocolli Salad
Cabbage & Mushroom Salad
Carrot & Beetroot Salad
Carrot & Broccoli Salad
Carrot & Kale Salad
Coconut Pickled Salad
Green Bean Salad
Jaw Dropping Tofu Burgers
Kale & Sprout Salad
Lentil & Kale Salad
Mixed Spice Pumpkin Soup
Moroccan Inspired Cabbage Salad
Pickle Pasta Salad
Potato & Avocado Salad
Potato & Kale Salad
Sauerkraut & Ricotta Salad
Spring Salad
Sweet Potato & Cabbage Salad
Sweet Potato Pasta Bake
Sweet Potato with Dried Fruit Salad
Sweet Potato, Spinach & Rice Salad
Tofu Chilli Salad
Vegetable Stir-Fry
Vitamin-Packed Spiced Soup

2.2.1 Bean & Sweet Potato Salad

Ingredients:
Zucchini (1/4 cup)
Mixed Beans (3/4 cup)
Sweet Potato (1 cup)
Carrot (1)
Corn (1/4 cup)
Garlic (1 clove)
Olive oil (to dress)

Preparation time:
15 minutes

Serves:
1

Nutrition friendly:
Gluten-Free
Vegan
Vegetarian

Guide:
Slice sweet potato into chunks – place in a microwave safe container and cook through (or, you may choose to cook on the stove top). Once cooked rinse with cold water and let it cool. Leaving the skin on slice the sweet potato into cubes.

Add carrot, zucchini and corn to the microwave safe dish (or stove top) – cook through and slice the carrot and zucchini into cubes *after* they are cooked through.

Drain mixed beans and rinse thoroughly.

Slice garlic finely – add to salad bowl along with all other ingredients.

Dress with olive oil and stir through.

Done!

Tag your salad on Topicthread to be added to our gallery!

2.2.2 Broccoli & Olive Pasta

Ingredients:
Pasta, gluten-free (1/2 cup)
Broccoli (2 stems)
Garlic (1 clove)
Olives, Black (1/4 cup)
Tomato (1)
Cabbage (1/2 cup)
Olive Oil (to serve)

Preparation time:
20 minutes

Serves:
1

Nutrition friendly:
Gluten-Free
Vegan
Vegetarian

Guide:
Place pasta on either stove top or into a microwave safe container to cook through. Let cool in bowl once done.
Slice broccoli and cabbage finely.
Slice tomato into cubes.
Finely slice olives and garlic.
Add ingredients to pasta bowl and lightly dress with olive oil.
Done!

Tag your pasta salad on Topicthread to be added to our gallery!

2.2.3 Cabbage & Beans

Ingredients:
Cabbage (1 cup)
Edamame Beans (1 cup)
Tomato (1)
Goats Cheese (30g)
Pickled Ginger (20g)
Mayonnaise (vegan friendly, or your preferred dressing)

Preparation time:
20 minutes

Serves:
1

Nutrition friendly:
Gluten-Free
Vegetarian

Guide:
Place edamame beans into bowl and pour boiling water over beans. Let sit until steamed lightly through.
Finely chop cabbage and place into salad bowl.
Chop tomato into cubes. Remove the seeds and place into the salad bowl.
Crumble goats cheese with your fingertips lightly over, placing into salad bowl.
Drain edamame beans and "pop" out individual beans into salad bowl.
Add pickled ginger to salad bowl and stir through ingredients before dressing with mayonnaise.
Done!

Tag your salad on Topicthread to be added to our gallery!

2.2.4 Cabbage & Mushroom Pasta Salad

Ingredients:
Pasta, Gluten-Free
(optional)
Cabbage (1/2 cup)
Mushrooms (1/2 cup)
Stuffed Olives (20g)
Pickled Ginger (20g)
Capsicum (1/4)
Diced Tomatoes (1
can)

Preparation time:
30 minutes

Serves:
1

Nutrition friendly:
Gluten-Free
Vegan
Vegetarian

Guide:
Bring water to boil and place pasta into saucepan – cook through until it has reached your desired texture.
Heat saucepan and add diced tomatoes – simmer until warm.
Slice mushrooms and add to saucepan of simmering tomatoes.
Slice cabbage finely and add to serving bowl.
Dice capsicum, finely cut olives and slice ginger before adding to serving bowl.
Once pasta is cooked through – drain, rinse and add to simmering saucepan.
Leave pasta to simmer until ingredients are nicely blended – add to serving bowl and stir through with other ingredients.
Done!

Tag your pasta salad on Topicthread to be added to our gallery!

2.2.5 Cabbage & Pickle Salad

Ingredients:
Cabbage (1 cup)
Tomatoes (1)
Ricotta (50g)
Dill Pickles (2)
Sauerkraut (handful)
Pepper (to season)

Preparation time:
15 minutes

Serves:
1

Nutrition friendly:
Gluten-Free
Vegetarian

Guide:
Finely chop cabbage – add to salad bowl.
Chop tomato into cubes – squeeze juices out lightly then add to salad bowl.
Slice pickles finely then add to salad bowl.
Chop sauerkraut into 2-3cm strips – add to salad bowl.
Crumble ricotta with your fingers into the salad bowl then lightly blend all ingredients together. Add pepper to serve.
Done!

Tag your salad on Topicthread to be added to our gallery!

2.2.6 Cabbage & Broccoli Salad

Ingredients:
Shallots (1 stem)
Cabbage (1 cup)
Chia Seeds (few sprinkles)
Sweet Potato (1/2 cup)
Broccoli (1 cup)
Beetroot (1/2 cup)
Olive Oil

Preparation time:
20 minutes

Serves:
1

Nutrition friendly:
Gluten-Free
Vegan
Vegetarian

Guide:
Chop sweet potato into manageable pieces and steam (microwave *or* stove top). Once cooked let cool. Leaving skin on proceed to chop sweet potato into cubes.
Slice shallots and cabbage finely.
Chop broccoli into edible pieces then slice beetroot into cubes.
Stir ingredients through and sprinkle with chia seeds then drizzle with olive oil.
Done!

Tag your salad on Topicthread to be added to our gallery!

2.2.7 Cabbage & Mushroom Salad

Ingredients:
Sugarloaf Cabbage (1 cup)
Chilli Olives (50g)
Ricotta (30g)
Mushrooms (3/4 cup)
Cucumber (1/4 cup)
Sauerkraut (handful)

Preparation time:
15 minutes

Serves:
1

Nutrition friendly:
Gluten-Free
Vegetarian

Guide:
To begin, cut your sugarloaf cabbage finely then add to your salad bowl.
Cut spice filled olives in quarters and add to salad bowl.
Lightly crumble the ricotta with your fingers into the salad bowl.
Cut mushrooms finely and then segment into quarters then add to salad bowl.
Add the sauerkraut to salad bowl after cutting into centimetre long strips.
Done!

Tag your salad on Topicthread to be added to our gallery!

2.2.8 Carrot & Beetroot Salad

Ingredients:
Garlic (1 clove)
Chia Seeds (few sprinkles)
Kale (2 stems)
Carrot (2)
Beetroot (1/3 cup)
Olive oil

Preparation time:
10 minutes

Serves:
1

Nutrition friendly:
Gluten-Free
Vegan
Vegetarian

Guide:
Cook (optional) carrots through. Once cooled slice into cubes and add to salad bowl.
Slice kale finely and add to salad bowl.
Chop beetroot into cubes and slice garlic finely.
Add all ingredients to salad bowl including a few sprinkles of chia seeds and drizzle of olive oil.
Done!

Tag your salad on Topicthread to be added to our gallery!

2.2.9 Carrot & Broccoli Salad

Ingredients:
Broccoli (stem)
Corn (1/4 cup)
Mushrooms (1/2 cup)
Carrots (1)
Lentils (1/2 cup)
Olive Oil

Preparation time:
15 minutes

Serves:
1

Nutrition friendly:
Gluten-Free
Vegan
Vegetarian

Guide:
Drain lentils and place into salad bowl.
Cook corn lightly on the stove top – place into salad bowl
once cooked through.
Slice mushrooms – add to salad bowl.
Chop carrots and broccoli into fine, edible pieces.
Stir ingredients – drizzle with olive oil.
Done!

Tag your salad on Topicthread to be added to our gallery!

2.2.10 Carrot & Kale Salad

Ingredients:
Kale (1 stem)
Beetroot (1/3 cup)
Chia Seeds (few sprinkles)
Carrot (1)
Sweet Potato (1/4cup)
Cabbage (1/2 cup)
Garlic (1 clove)
Avocado (1/2)
Olive Oil

Preparation time:
15 minutes

Serves:
1

Nutrition friendly:
Gluten-Free
Vegan
Vegetarian

Guide:
Chop sweet potato into cubes and steam (microwave *or* stove top) – set aside to cool.
Slice kale and cabbage finely.
Chop beetroot, avocado and carrot into cubes.
Slice garlic finely and add to salad bowl along with all other ingredients.
Stir through ingredients and dress with chia seeds and olive oil.
Done!

Tag your salad on Topicthread to be added to our gallery!

2.2.11 Coconut Pickled Salad

Ingredients:
Fresh Coconut (1/2 cup)
Dill Pickles (2)
Tomato (1)
Cabbage (1/2 cup)
Spinach (50g)
Grated Cheese (20g)

Preparation time:
15 minutes

Serves:
1

Nutrition friendly:
Gluten-Free
Vegetarian

Guide:
Open fresh coconut and peel away "inside" of coconut
until you have filled ½ cup (prepacked, optional).
Slice pickles finely.
Chop tomato into cubes then finely slice cabbage.
Pull a part spinach lightly then add to salad bowl along
with all other ingredients.
Stir through ingredients and add grated cheese to serve.
Done!

Tag your salad on Topicthread to be added to our gallery!

2.2.12 Green Bean Salad

Ingredients:

Green Beans (1 ½ cups)
Fresh Spinach (30g)
Mushrooms (30g)
Capsicum (1/4)
Fetta (30g)
Sundried Tomatoes (30g)
Cabbage (1/4 cup)
Garlic Infused Stuffed Olives (30g)
Cucumber (1/4 cup)
Celery Sticks (1)

Preparation time:
20 minutes

Serves:
1

Nutrition friendly:
Gluten-Free
Vegetarian

Guide:
Cut beans into inch-length pieces (steam, optional) – add to salad bowl.
Chop cucumber and celery into cube-like pieces – add to salad bowl.
Tear spinach into halves and add to salad bowl.
Chop sundried tomato pieces into strips – add to salad bowl.
Slice cabbage and mushrooms finely then add to salad bowl.
Chop capsicum into cubes then cut olives into halves – add to salad bowl.
Crumble fetta using your fingers, into salad bowl and lightly stir ingredients together.
Done!

Tag your salad on Topicthread to be added to our gallery!

2.2.13 Jaw Dropping Tofu Burgers

Ingredients:

Burger:
Bread roll of your
choice (gluten-free
optional)
Spinach (20g)
Tomato (1)
Mozzarella Cheese
(handful)
Pineapple (20g)
Pickled Ginger (10g)
Mushroom (20g)
Aioli Sauce (to dress)

Seasoned tofu:
Tofu (30g, meat
substitution optional)
Chilli Flakes (1
teaspoon)
Minced Garlic (1
teaspoon)
Minced Ginger (1
teaspoon)
Parsley (1 teaspoon)
Soy Sauce (1 teaspoon)

Preparation time:
30 minutes

Serves:
1

Nutrition friendly:
Vegetarian

Guide:
To make tofu patties, carefully slice patty sized portion
from the tofu and set aside on paper towel to soak up
excess water. Stir *all* seasoned tofu ingredients together in
a bowl.
Once ingredients are ready, place tofu patty into marinade
and let sit before placing into low-heat saucepan.
Add the marinade to the saucepan with the patty to allow
the ingredients to further soak into the patty.
Simmer for 5-10 minutes and then set aside.
To make the burger bun, simply cut your bread roll into
halves and begin to add the ingredients.

Place spinach onto bread roll, followed by the tomato and mushrooms.

Add your tofu patty to the bread roll and then add the mozzarella cheese on top, allowing it to slightly melt from the heat of the patty.

Lastly, add the pineapple, ginger then top with aioli sauce.
Done!

Tag your tofu burger on Topicthread to be added to our gallery!

2.2.14 Kale & Sprout Salad

Ingredients:
Kale (2 stems)
Sweet Potato (1/2 cup)
Bean Sprouts (1 cup)
Avocado (1/2)
Carrot (1/2)
Celery (1)
Olive Oil

Preparation time:
15 minutes

Serves:
1

Nutrition friendly:
Gluten-Free
Vegan
Vegetarian

Guide:
Chop sweet potato into manageable pieces to steam –
cook through and set aside to cool. Once cooled chop into
cubes.
Slice kale and celery.
Chop carrot and avocado into cubes.
Add bean sprouts to salad bowl along with all other
ingredients.
Stir all ingredients through then drizzle with olive oil.
Done!

Tag your salad on Topicthread to be added to our gallery!

2.2.15 Lentil & Kale Salad

Ingredients:
Kale (2 stems)
Beetroot (1/2 cup)
Lentils (1 cup)
Tomato (1)
Mayonnaise (Vegan Friendly, to serve)

Preparation time:
10 minutes

Serves:
1

Nutrition friendly:
Gluten-Free
Vegan
Vegetarian

Guide:
Rinse lentils from your preference of pre-cooked cans; if
you would like to cook your own, bring to boil and cook
until ready to serve, remembering to rinse thoroughly.
Slice tomato and beetroot into cubes.
Chop kale finely – add all ingredients to salad bowl.
Lightly drizzle with your choice of dressing – mayonnaise
suggested.
Done!

Tag your salad on Topicthread to be added to our gallery!

2.2.16 Mixed Spice Pumpkin Soup

Ingredients:
Pumpkin (1/4 of a whole)
Natural Yoghurt (50ml)
Pepper (1 teaspoon)
Garlic powder (1 teaspoon)
Chilli Flakes (1 teaspoon)

Preparation time:
30 minutes

Serves:
4

Nutrition friendly:
Gluten-Free
Vegetarian

Guide:
Chop pumpkin into medium sized pieces (leave skin on).
Bring water to boil in large saucepan – add pumpkin pieces.
Let the pumpkin cook through until nice and soft – drain with cold water.
Once pumpkin has cooled peel off the skin.
Add pumpkin to blender, ensuring the pumpkin has cooled.
Blend pumpkin until nice and smooth.
Pour pumpkin back into saucepan and lightly simmer – heating the soup.
Add yoghurt and spices to soup – stir through and simmer until desired consistency has been reached.
Done!

Tag your soup on Topicthread to be added to our gallery!

2.2.17 Moroccan Inspired Cabbage Salad

Ingredients:
Sugarloaf Cabbage (1 cup)
Mushrooms (50g)
Moroccan Chilli Olives (50g)
Dill Pickles (2)
Sauerkraut (20g)
Cucumber (1/4)
Capsicum (1/4)
Ricotta (30g)
Tomato (1)

Preparation time:
20 minutes

Serves:
1

Nutrition friendly:
Gluten-Free
Vegetarian

Guide:
Chop sugarloaf cabbage finely.
Slice mushrooms, pickles and olives finely.
Chop sauerkraut to ensure any "long" strips are shortened.
Cut cucumber lengthways and then into cubes.
Chop capsicum and tomato into cubes.
Mix all ingredients into a large salad bowl.
Before serving, add the ricotta. Crumble ricotta gently with your fingers into salad and then use your hands to mix through.
Done!

Tag your salad on Topicthread to be added to our gallery!

2.2.18 Pickle Pasta Salad

Ingredients:
Dill Pickles (2)
Sauerkraut (handful)
Spinach (30g)
Tomato (1)
Pasta, Gluten-Free (optional, ½ cup)
Garlic (1 clove)
Olive Oil (to serve)

Preparation time:
20 minutes

Serves:
1

Nutrition friendly:
Gluten-Free
Vegan
Vegetarian

Guide:
Bring water to boil and cook pasta until it has reached your preferred level of consistency. Drain and rinse with cold water.
Pull a part spinach (fresh) and slice sauerkraut into edible pieces.
Chop tomato into cubes.
Slice pickles and garlic finely – add to salad bowl along with all other ingredient.
Drizzle with olive oil.
Done!

Tag your pasta salad on Topicthread to be added to our gallery!

2.2.19 Potato & Avocado Salad

Ingredients:
Beetroot (1/4 cup)
Avocado (1/2)
Chia Seeds (few sprinkles)
Garlic (1 clove)
Carrot (1/4)
Potato (2 small)
Cabbage (1/2 cup)

Preparation time:
20 minutes

Serves:
1

Nutrition friendly:
Gluten-Free
Vegan
Vegetarian

Guide:
Chop potato into cubes and steam until cooked through.
Once cooked, rinse and place into salad bowl.
Slice cabbage and place into salad bowl.
Chop beetroot, avocado and carrot into cubes – add to salad bowl
Finely slice garlic and add to salad bowl, stirring through all ingredients before lastly adding the chia seeds.
Done!

Tag your salad on Topicthread to be added to our gallery!

2.2.20 Potato & Kale Salad

Ingredients:
Kale (1 stem)
Beetroot (1/2 cup)
Carrot (1)
Potato (2 small)
Mayonnaise (vegan friendly)

Preparation time:
15 minutes

Serves:
1

Nutrition friendly:
Gluten-Free
Vegan
Vegetarian

Guide:
Chop potato up into cubes – cook through in microwave (or stove top). Once cooked, set aside to cool.
Chop carrot into cubes – cook through in microwave (or stove top). Once cooked, set aside to cool (note: potato *and* carrots can be cooked together).
Chop beetroot into cubes.
Finely pull a part kale – add to salad bowl along with all other ingredients.
Stir through and dress with mayonnaise.
Done!

Tag your salad on Topicthread to be added to our gallery!

2.2.21 Sauerkraut & Ricotta Salad

Ingredients:
Sauerkraut (40g)
Ricotta (40g)
Dill Pickles (2)
Moroccan Spiced Stuffed Olives (30g)

Preparation time:
15 minutes

Serves:
1

Nutrition friendly:
Gluten-Free
Vegetarian

Guide:
Cut sauerkraut into inch-long pieces – add to bowl.
Slice pickles finely – add to bowl.
Chop olives into quarters and add to bowl along with its accompanying dressing.
Crumble ricotta using your fingers over bowl.
Lightly stir ingredients through salad bowl with your fingers.
Done!

Tag your salad on Topicthread to be added to our gallery!

2.2.22 Spring Salad

Ingredients:
Broccoli (1 stem)
Cabbage (1/2 cup)
Tomato (1)
Dill Pickle (1)
Pickled Ginger (20g)
Mushrooms (30g)
Grated Cheese, handful

Preparation time:
15 minutes

Serves:
1

Nutrition friendly:
Gluten-Free
Vegetarian

Guide:
Slice broccoli, cabbage and mushrooms roughly.
Chop tomato into cubes.
Slice pickles and ginger finely.
Add all ingredients to salad bowl, stir through and add grated cheese.
Done!

Tag your salad on Topicthread to be added to our gallery!

2.2.23 Sweet Potato & Cabbage Salad

Ingredients:
Sweet Potato (1 cup)
Avocado (1/2)
Carrot (1)
Chia Seeds (few sprinkles)
Cabbage (1/4 cup)
Ginger (centimetre)
Garlic (1 clove)
Olive Oil

Preparation time:
20 minutes

Serves:
1

Nutrition friendly:
Gluten-Free
Vegan
Vegetarian

Guide:
Chop sweet potato roughly and steam. Once cooked through, allow time to cool then proceed to cut into edible sized pieces.
Chop carrots and cabbage roughly.
Slice avocado finely then slice garlic and ginger.
Add all ingredients to salad bowl and sprinkle with chia seeds.
Stir ingredients through and drizzle with olive oil.
Done!

Tag your salad on Topicthread to be added to our gallery!

2.2.24 Sweet Potato Pasta Bake

Ingredients:

Sweet Potato (1 ½ cups)
Pasta, Gluten-Free (optional, 1 ½ cups))
Spinach (80g)

Tomatoes (2)
Mushrooms (50g)
Ricotta (30g)
Grated Cheese (30g)

Preparation time:
60 minutes

Serves:
6

Nutrition friendly:
Gluten-Free
Vegetarian

Guide:
Set oven to 180C to preheat.
Bring water to boil and cook pasta until done to your choice of consistency. Drain and set aside.
Chop sweet potato into manageable pieces – cook through using the microwave *or* stove top. Set aside to cool. Once cooled chop cubes.
Tear apart spinach into desired pieces and add to pasta.
Slice mushrooms finely and add to pasta.
Chop tomatoes into cubes – add to pasta.
Stir through ricotta into the pasta and mix through all ingredients.
Add sweet potato to pasta and stir through.
Place into baking dish and top with grated cheese.
Proceed to place baking dish into over and let bake through until cheese has melted nicely (20-30minutes).
Done!

Tag your salad on Topicthread to be added to our gallery!

2.2.25 Sweet Potato with Dried Fruit Salad

Ingredients:
Dried Fruit (1/4 cup, Prunes suggested)
Capsicum (1/2)
Beetroot (1/4 cup)
Sweet Potato (1 cup)
Carrots (1)
Kale (1 stem)
Mayonnaise (vegan friendly)

Preparation time:
20 minutes

Serves:
1

Nutrition friendly:
Gluten-Free
Vegan
Vegetarian

Guide:
Chop sweet potato into manageable pieces and steam – using the microwave or using the stove top. Once cooked let cool then chop into cubes, leaving the skin on.
Slice capsicum and beetroot into cubes.
Chop carrots into cubes (steaming optional).
Slice kale finely – add to salad bowl along with all other ingredients. If using prunes, slice finely before adding.
Stir ingredients through then add mayonnaise to dress.
Done!

Tag your salad on Topicthread to be added to our gallery!

2.2.26 Sweet Potato, Spinach & Rice Salad

Ingredients:
Sweet Potato (1 cup)
Mushrooms (50g)
Fetta (30g)
Tomato (1)
Fresh Spinach (40g)
Sauerkraut (20g)
Ginger (1 teaspoon)
Rice (1/4 cup)
Corn, Peas, Beans (1/2 cup combined)

Preparation time:
30 minutes

Serves:
1

Nutrition friendly:
Gluten-Free
Vegan
Vegetarian

Guide:
Chop sweet potato into manageable pieces then steam (microwave *or* stove top).
Steam rice and cook through until done.
Steam corn, peas and beans together (microwave or stove top). Once all steaming is finished, set aside all ingredients.
Slice mushrooms finely. Chop tomatoes into cubes, squeezing juices out lightly before adding to salad bowl. Tear spinach with your fingers into halves and add to salad bowl. Chop sauerkraut into shortened pieces. Once cooled, chop sweet potato into cubes and add to salad bowl along with all other ingredients.

Slice ginger finely and add to salad bowl. Crumble fetta through fingertips into salad bowl.
Mix all ingredients through with fingertips.
Done!

Tag your rice salad on Topicthread to be added to our gallery!

2.2.27 Tofu Chilli Salad

Ingredients:
Tomato (1)
Edamame Beans (50g)
Sauerkraut (handful)
Cucumber (1/4 cup)
Capsicum (1/4)
Spinach (30g)
Carrot (1/2)
Stuffed Olives (20g)
Tofu (70g)
Mushrooms (50g)
For the Marinade:
Minced Ginger (1 teaspoon)
Minced Garlic (1 teaspoon)
Lemon Juice (1 teaspoon)
Salt and Pepper (to taste)
Masala (1 teaspoon)

Preparation time:
30 minutes

Serves:
1

Nutrition friendly:
Gluten-Free
Vegan
Vegetarian

Guide:
To make marinade, combine ginger, garlic, lemon juice, salt, pepper and masala to *your* taste.
Slice tofu into cubes and then place into marinade. Allow the tofu to rest in marinade (option: lightly cook through in heated frypan).

Steam edamame beans lightly. Pop beans out of their shoots then add to salad bowl.

Add sauerkraut to serving bowl being careful to "cut" longer pieces into lengths no more than 2-3 centimetres.

Chop cucumber into cubes and place into serving bowl.

Cut capsicum and carrot into cubes then add to serving bowl.

Slice mushrooms and olives finely then add to serving bowl.

Lastly, add the now marinated tofu to the serving bowl along with the remainder of the marinade to lightly dress all ingredients. Stir through all ingredients before serving.

Done!

Tag your salad on Topicthread to be added to our gallery!

2.2.28 Vegetable Stir-Fry

Ingredients:
Mushrooms (1 cup)
Broccolini (1 stem/bunch)
Cabbage (1 cup)
Spiced Olives (20g)
Tomatoes (1)
Salt and Pepper (to season)

Preparation time:
20 minutes

Serves:
1

Nutrition friendly:
Gluten-Free
Vegan
Vegetarian

Guide:
Slice mushrooms finely and add to wok.
Chop broccolini into edible pieces – add to wok.
Slice cabbage finely – add to wok.
Bring wok to heat and add a pinch of water to help ingredients cook through.
Add a pinch of olive oil when almost done.
Turn wok off.
Slice tomatoes into cubes and olives into quarters – add to wok.
Add salt and pepper and stir through ingredients.
Done!

Tag your stir-fry on Topicthread to be added to our gallery!

2.2.29 Vitamin-Packed Spiced Soup

Ingredients:
Pumpkin (4 cups, blended)
Spinach (2 cups, blended)
Cabbage (1 cup, blended)
Natural Yoghurt (200ml)
Garlic Salt (1 tablespoon)
Salt (1 teaspoon)
Chilli Powder (1 tablespoon)
Pepper (1 teaspoon)
Chicken Stock (1 teaspoon)

Preparation time:
75 minutes

Serves:
8

Nutrition friendly:
Vegetarian

Guide:
Bring saucepan to boil.
Chop pumpkin into medium pieces and place in saucepan (leaving the skin on).
Cook pumpkin through until nice and soft. Take off the heat and rinse with cold water to cool. Once pumpkin has cooled peel skin off then place into blender.
Blend pumpkin until smooth then add back to saucepan.
Add fresh spinach straight into blender – blend until nice and smooth. Add blended spinach to saucepan.
Place cabbage (chopped) into blender and blend until smooth – add to saucepan.
Bring saucepan to heat and lightly simmer – stirring through ingredients. Add spices and stock flavour (optional) to saucepan and stir through.

Lastly, add yoghurt to reach desired consistency and taste
– stir through.
Done!

Tag your soup on Topicthread to be added to our gallery!

2.3 Snacks – Muffins

To keep our metabolisms honest and up to speed, we need to eat. When we eat our metabolism kicks into gear to "digest" what we are eating, turning our food sources into energy. By regularly feeding our metabolism it remains alert and is more readily able to convert our food into energy sources.

There's more to it. Without overcomplicating the premise here, which is to outline the benefits associated with "snacking" – our metabolism has an optimal rate of functioning. This "rate" as such aligns with the energy we require on a daily basis. In short, if we consume more "energy" than we require, our metabolism becomes sluggish. And when our metabolism becomes sluggish it isn't as efficient at converting our food to energy – it takes longer, and instead of converting our food to energy, it does what we don't want – it is stored. What many may be surprised to learn here is that it works both ways – if we don't regularly feed our metabolism, regardless of "what" we are eating, it too becomes inefficient.

In order to optimize our metabolism, it is recommended to eat regularly – consistent meals throughout the day. This means, rather than eating larger portions typically three times a day, it is in fact encouraged to snack between meals which then reduces the amounts our metabolism has to break-down at meal time. Essentially, your three meals are key, and the meals in between are stimulators to keep your metabolism honest.

Featured Recipes:

Banana & Rasberry Forest Muffins (Cake)
Banana & Oat Muffins
Banana, Oat & Choc-Chip Muffins
Beetroot & Kale Muffins
Choc-Banana Muffins (Bread)
Cocoa & Chia Muffins
Pumpkin, Zucchini & Carrot Muffins
Super C Muffins
Superfood Muffins
Sweet Potato, Chia & Kale Muffins
Vanilla Apple Muffin

Being mindful of keeping our metabolisms honest, 2.3 and 2.4 will provide quick and easy snacks that are packed with fruits and/or vegetables – but also flavoursome! These include sweet and savoury muffins (2.3) along with a combination of quick and easy go-to smoothies (2.4). The best part? All snacks can easily be made vegan *and* gluten-free, if not already, through simple substitutions, whilst remaining vegetarian friendly.

2.3.1 Banana & Raspberry Forest Muffins (Cake)

Ingredients:
Bananas (3)
Raspberries (2 cups)
Cocoa Powder (1 tablespoon)
Cinnamon (1 tablespoon)
Vanilla Essence (2 tablespoons)
Eggs (2)
Self-Raising Flour (1 ½ cups)
Milk (3/4 cup)
Chocolate (100g to melt, 50g to Grate)

Preparation time:
60 minutes + 15 minutes preparation

Serves:
12

Nutrition friendly:
Vegetarian

Guide:
Preheat Oven to 180C.
Mash bananas into mixing bowl until smooth consistency has formed.
Add raspberries to mixing bowl along with the cocoa powder, cinnamon and vanilla essence – stir through.
Add self-raising flour slowly along with the milk. Once the desired consistency has been reached, mix through the eggs and stir until desired texture has been reached.
Place mixture into your choice of muffin tin or cake tray (pictured).
Place in over at 180C for 60 minutes – checking after 45 minutes and then every 5 minutes to ensure baking consistency.

Melt chocolate over stove top (by boiling water and placing metal bowl on top) – allow chocolate to melt to smooth consistency and let sit.

Grate chocolate and leave in refrigerator.

Once muffins (or cake) has cooked through let cool on baking rack then proceed to add the melted chocolate – coating the top layer then let cool.

Once muffins (or cake) has cooled, lastly add the grated chocolate over the top.

Done!

Tag your muffin on Topicthread to be added to our gallery!

2.3.2 Banana & Oat Muffins

Ingredients:
Bananas (6)
Chia Seeds (handful)
Oats (1 cup)
Self-Raising Flour (1 cup)
Soy Milk (1 cup)

Preparation time:
60 minutes + 15 minutes preparation

Serves:
6

Nutrition friendly:
Vegan
Vegetarian

Guide:
Preheat oven to 180C.
Mash bananas through until smooth texture has been reached.
Place mashed banana in mixing bowl and add the chia seeds and oats – stir together.
Add the self-raising flour and soy milk to mixing bowl – stir until reached a smooth consistency.
Prepare muffin tins or baking tray of your choice.
Place in over at 180C for 60 minutes – checking after 30 minutes and then every 10 minutes to ensure baking consistency.
Done!

Tag your muffin on Topicthread to be added to our gallery!

2.3.3 Banana, Oat & Choc-Chip Muffins

Ingredients:
Bananas (4)
Oats (1/2 cup)
Self-Raising Flour (1/2 cup)
Soy Milk (1/4 cup)
Cinnamon (1 tablespoon)

Preparation time:
40 minutes + 10 minutes preparation

Serves:
12

Nutrition friendly:
Vegan
Vegetarian

Guide:
Pre-heat oven to 180C.
Mash bananas inside a mixing bowl until smooth consistency has been reached.
Place oats and flour into mixing bowl – stir through until desired consistency formed.
Stir through milk until you have formed a nice texture.
Add the cinnamon and give a final stir of all ingredients.
Place mixture into muffin tray and evenly distribute.
It's now time to place your tray into the oven. Set timer for 40 minutes. Check on muffins frequently to ensure oven is working "with" your mixture, and not against!
Once your 40 minutes are up, set aside muffins to cool and then empty onto cooling rack.
Done!

Tag your muffin on Topicthread to be added to our gallery!

2.3.4 Beetroot & Kale Muffins

Ingredients:
Beetroot (1 cup)
Kale (3 stems)
Self-Raising Flour (2 cups)
Milk (2 cups)
Eggs (2)

Preparation time:
60 minutes baking + 20 minutes preparation

Serves:
8

Nutrition friendly:
Vegetarian

Guide:
Preheat oven to 180C.
Slice beetroot into small cube pieces and add to mixing bowl being careful not to add "too much" liquid. You have the option to add "a little" liquid and reduce the amount of milk you choose to add.
Slice the kale up finely and add to mixing bowl.
Add the self-raising flour, milk and eggs to mixing bowl – stir until reached a smooth consistency.
Prepare muffin tins or baking tray of your choice.
Place in oven at 180C for 60 minutes – checking after 30 minutes and then every 10 minutes to ensure baking consistency.
Done!

Tag your muffin on Topicthread to be added to our gallery!

2.3.5 Choc-Banana Muffins (Bread)

Ingredients:
Bananas (3)
Gluten Free Flour (1 cup, optional)
Milk (1/2 cup)
Mixed Spice (1 tablespoon)
Chocolate (50g)

Preparation time:
45 minutes + 15 minutes preparation

Serves:
6

Nutrition friendly:
Gluten-Free
Vegetarian

Guide:
Preheat oven to 180C.
Mash bananas into mixing bowl until they have reached a smooth consistency.
Add flour and milk progressively until the mixture has formed a nice texture.
Proceed to add the mixed spice and stir through thoroughly.
Break chocolate up into small "chunks" and stir into the mixture.
Prepare muffin tins or baking tray (pictured) of your choice.
Place in over at 180C for 45 minutes – checking after 30 minutes and then every 10 minutes to ensure baking consistency.
Done!

Tag your muffin on Topicthread to be added to our gallery!

2.3.6 Cocoa & Chia Muffins

Ingredients:
Chia seeds (handful)
Cacao (1/4 cup)
Sugar (1/2 cup)
Self-Raising Flour (1 1/4 cup)
Vanilla Essence (1 tablespoon)
Egg (1)
Milk (1 cup)

Preparation time:
40 minutes + 10 minutes preparation

Serves:
8

Nutrition friendly:
Vegetarian

Guide:
Add the self-raising flour, milk and eggs to mixing bowl –
stir until reached a smooth consistency.
Add cacao, chia seeds, sugar and vanilla essence, one at a
time to the mixing bowl, stirring until a smooth
consistency has been reached.
Prepare muffin tins or baking tray of your choice.
Place in oven at 180C for 40 minutes – checking after 30
minutes and then every 5 minutes to ensure baking
consistency.
Done!

Tag your muffin on Topicthread to be added to our gallery!

2.3.7 Pumpkin, Zucchini & Carrot Muffins

Ingredients (family size):
Pumpkin (400g)
Zucchini (4)
Carrot (4)
Beetroot Juice (250ml)
Mixed Spice (1 tablespoon)
Eggs (4)
Plain Flour (2 ¼ cups)
Milk (1/2 cup)

Preparation time:
45 minutes + 20 minutes preparation

Serves:
18

Nutrition friendly:
Vegetarian

Guide:
Pre-heat oven to 180C.
Peel pumpkin and cut into pieces ready to grate.
Wash carrots and zucchinis then proceed to grate
pumpkin, carrots and zucchini directly into mixing bowl.
Add eggs and stir through. Your mixture will be nice and
moist now - add the flour slowly until your mixture
reaches a good consistency then stop.
Add the milk and beetroot juice slowly whilst adding the
remaining flour as necessary.
Add the mixed spice and stir through.
Use baking trays of your choice. Muffin trays are
recommended.
Place mixture into muffin tin and evenly distribute.
It's now time to place your tray into the oven. Set timer for
45 minutes. Check on muffins frequently to ensure oven is
working "with" your mixture, and not against!

Once your 45 minutes are up, set aside muffins to cool
and then empty onto cooling rack.
Done!

Tag your muffin on Topicthread to be added to our gallery!

2.3.8 Super C Muffins

Ingredients:
Self-Raising Flour (1 cup)
Caster Sugar (1/4 cup)
Cacao (1/4 cup)
Chia Seeds (handful)
Carrots (3)
Vanilla Essence (1 tablespoon)
Milk (1 cup)
Eggs (2)

Preparation time:
60 minutes + 20 minutes preparation

Serves:
8

Nutrition friendly:
Vegetarian

Guide:
Preheat oven to 180C.
Finely grate carrots (peeling optional, ensure to rinse).
Add the self-raising flour, milk and eggs to mixing bowl –
stir until reached a smooth consistency.
Add the cater sugar, vanilla essence, chia seeds and cacao
powder and stir through until mixture is smooth.
Prepare muffin tins or baking tray of your choice.
Place in oven at 180C for 60 minutes – checking after 30
minutes and then every 10 minutes to ensure baking
consistency.
Done!

Tag your muffin on Topicthread to be added to our gallery!

2.3.9 Superfood Muffins

Ingredients:

Self-Raising Flour (1 cup)
Egg (1)
Milk (1 cup)
Vanilla Essence (1 tablespoon)

Bunch Kale (1 Cup)
Cacao (1/4 cup)
Chia Seeds (handful)
Oats (1 cup)
Bananas (3, ripe)
Butter (1/2 cup)

Preparation time:
60 minutes + 20 minutes preparation

Serves:
8

Nutrition friendly:
Vegetarian

Guide:
Preheat oven to 180C.
Mash bananas in mixing bowl until they have reached a smooth texture.
Slice the kale finely and then add to mixing bowl.
Add oats, chia seeds and cacao to mixing bowl and stir through ingredients.
Then proceed to add self-raising flour, milk, eggs, butter (melted) and vanilla essence – one at a time, stirring through to ensure all ingredients are nicely blended.
Prepare muffin tins or baking tray of your choice.
Place in oven at 180C for 60 minutes – checking after 30 minutes and then every 10 minutes to ensure baking consistency.
Done!

Tag your muffin on Topicthread to be added to our gallery!

2.3.10 Sweet Potato, Chia & Kale Muffins

Ingredients:
Kale (2 cups)
Sweet Potato (2 ½ cups, mashed)
Chia Seeds (handful)
Self-Raising Flour (1 cup)
Milk (1 cup)
Eggs (2)

Preparation time:
60 minutes + 20 minutes preparation time

Serves:
8

Nutrition friendly:
Vegetarian

Guide:
Preheat oven to 180C.
Steam sweet potato until tender. Rinse with cold water and let cool. Once cooled, mash through then add to mixing bowl.
Slice the kale up finely and add to mixing bowl.
Add the self-raising flour, milk and eggs to mixing bowl – stir until reached a smooth consistency.
Add chia seeds to mixing bowl and give it a final stir through.
Prepare muffin tins or baking tray of your choice.
Place in oven at 180C for 60 minutes – checking after 30 minutes and then every 10 minutes to ensure baking consistency.
Done!

Tag your muffin on Topicthread to be added to our gallery!

2.3.11 Vanilla Apple Muffins

Ingredients:
Apples (2)
Vanilla Essence (1 tablespoon)
Cinnamon (2 tablespoons)
Self-Raising Flour (1 ½ cups)
Milk (1 ½ cups)
Eggs (2)

Preparation time:
60 minutes baking + 20 minutes preparation

Serves:
6

Nutrition friendly:
Vegetarian

Guide:
Preheat oven to 180C.
Chop apples finely into small cubes (peel is optional).
Add the self-raising flour, milk and eggs to mixing bowl –
stir until reached a smooth consistency.
Add the vanilla essence and cinnamon to the mixing bowl
– stir until mixed through.
Prepare muffin tins or baking tray of your choice.
Place in oven at 180C for 60 minutes – checking after 30
minutes and then every 10 minutes to ensure baking
consistency.
Done!

Tag your muffin on Topicthread to be added to our gallery!

2.4 Snacks – Smoothies

It is well known that we *should* be getting "this many" fruits and "that many" vegetables in our diet, every day. Yet somehow, what we eat never seems enough! When eating nutritious meals that appear jam-packed with vitamins and minerals, which 2.2 presented, sometimes this doesn't always go to plan. In order to keep the "keys" to restoring and regaining your *optimal wellbeing*, your *own* individual gut health is priority.

Time is one of the biggest factors that cause disruption when working towards taking control of your health *and* fitness. Right now I am letting you know that I understand – I get it – this is thoroughly acknowledged and is why 2.4 herein presents simplified smoothies that are incredibly *time* efficient and flavoursome. These smoothies form a part of your Guide to be used as snacks between meals, keeping you honest in the transition between regaining your renewed lifestyle.

Featured Recipes:

Banana & Blueberry Smoothie
Banana & Mixed Berry Smoothie
Banana & Rasberry Smoothie
Banana & Strawberry Smoothie
Banana Smoothie
Manago, Pineapple & Strawberry Smoothie
Mango & Banana Smoothie
Orange & Pineapple Smoothie
Pineapple & Banana Smoothie
Strawberry, Blueberry & Banana Smoothie
Watermelon Smoothie

2.4.1 Banana & Blueberry Smoothie

Ingredients:
Banana (1)
Blueberries (1/2 cup)
Water (200ml)

Preparation time:
5 minutes

Serves:
1

Nutrition friendly:
Raw
Gluten-Free
Vegan
Vegetarian

Guide:
Chop banana into quarters – add to blender.
Add blueberries directly to blender.
Add water – blend away!
Done!

Tag your smoothie on Topicthread to be added to our gallery!

2.4.2 Banana & Mixed Berry Smoothie

Ingredients:
Banana (1)
Blueberries (1/4 cup)
Raspberries (1/4 cup)
Water (200ml)

Preparation time:
5 minutes

Serves:
1

Nutrition friendly:
Raw
Gluten-Free
Vegan
Vegetarian

Guide:
Chop banana into quarters – add to blender.
Add blueberries and raspberries directly into blender.
Add water – blend away!
Done!

Tag your smoothie on Topicthread to be added to our gallery!

2.4.3 Banana & Raspberry Smoothie

Ingredients:
Banana (1)
Raspberries (1/2 cup)
Water (200ml)

Preparation time:
5 minutes

Serves:
1

Nutrition friendly:
Raw
Gluten-Free
Vegan
Vegetarian

Guide:
Chop banana into quarters – add to blender.
Add raspberries directly to blender.
Add water – blend away!
Done!

Tag your smoothie on Topicthread to be added to our gallery!

2.4.4 Banana & Strawberry Smoothie

Ingredients:
Banana (1)
Strawberries (1/2 cup)
Water (200ml)

Preparation time:
5 minutes

Serves:
1

Nutrition friendly:
Raw
Gluten-Free
Vegan
Vegetarian

Guide:
Chop banana into quarters – add to blender.
Slice strawberries in half – add to blender.
Add water - blend away!
Done!

Tag your smoothie on Topicthread to be added to our gallery!

2.4.5 Banana Smoothie

Ingredients:
Banana (1)
Water (200ml)

Preparation time:
5 minutes

Serves:
1

Nutrition friendly:
Raw
Gluten-Free
Vegan
Vegetarian

Guide:
Chop banana into quarters – add to blender.
Add water – blend away!
Done!

Tag your smoothie on Topicthread to be added to our gallery!

2.4.6 Mango, Pineapple & Strawberry Smoothie

Ingredients:
Mango (1/2 cup)
Pineapple (1/2 cup)
Strawberries (1/2 cup)
Water (200ml)

Preparation time:
5 minutes

Serves:
1

Nutrition friendly:
Raw
Gluten-Free
Vegan
Vegetarian

Guide:
Chop mango and pineapple into cubes – add to blender.
Slice strawberries in half – add to blender.
Add water – blend away!
Done!

Tag your smoothie on Topicthread to be added to our gallery!

2.4.7 Mango & Banana Smoothie

Ingredients:
Banana (1)
Mango (3/4 cup)
Water (200ml)

Preparation time:
5 minutes

Serves:
1

Nutrition friendly:
Raw
Gluten-Free
Vegan
Vegetarian

Guide:
Slice mango into cubes – add to blender.
Chop banana into quarters – add to blender.
Add water – blend away!
Done!

Tag your smoothie on Topicthread to be added to our gallery!

2.4.8 Orange & Pineapple Smoothie

Ingredients:
Oranges (2)
Pineapple (1 cup, sliced)
Water (150ml)

Preparation time:
5 minutes

Serves:
1

Nutrition friendly:
Raw
Gluten-Free
Vegan
Vegetarian

Guide:
Slice oranges into quarters, removing peel – add to blender.
Chop pineapple into manageable pieces – add to blender.
Add water – blend away!
Done!

Tag your smoothie on Topicthread to be added to our gallery!

2.4.9 Pineapple & Banana Smoothie

Ingredients:
Banana (1)
Pineapple (1 cup, sliced)
Water (200ml)

Preparation time:
5 minutes

Serves:
1

Nutrition friendly:
Raw
Gluten-Free
Vegan
Vegetarian

Guide:
Slice pineapple into cubes – add to blender.
Chop banana into quarters – add to blender.
Add water – blend away!
Done!

Tag your smoothie on Topicthread to be added to our gallery!

2.4.10 Strawberry, Blueberry & Banana Smoothie

Ingredients:
Banana (1)
Strawberries (1/4 cup)
Blueberries (1/4 cup)
Water (200ml)

Preparation time:
5 minutes

Serves:
1

Nutrition friendly:
Raw
Gluten-Free
Vegan
Vegetarian

Guide:
Slice strawberries in half - add to blender.
Chop banana into quarters – add to blender.
Add blueberries directly to blender.
Add water – blend away!
Done!

Tag your smoothie on Topicthread to be added to our gallery!

2.4.11 Watermelon Smoothie

Ingredients:
Watermelon (2 cups, sliced)
Banana (1)
Water (50ml)

Preparation time:
5 minutes

Serves:
1

Nutrition friendly:
Raw
Gluten-Free
Vegan
Vegetarian

Guide:
Slice watermelon into cubes – add to blender.
Chop banana into quarters – add to blender.
Add water – blend away!
Done!

Tag your smoothie on Topicthread to be added to our gallery!

2.5 Chicken, Fish, Beef or Lamb

Once upon a time, the stereotypical meal at dinner time was quite simply, *"meat and three vege"* – a colloquial phrase representative of a household staple in Australia. As too was for the lunchbox, including "meat sandwiches" alongside additional snacks and juices. The typical nutrition of the average person is inclusive of meat-based meals and snacks, plus an assortment of foods that fall under the "processed" category. Simply put, *meat* is a staple in the "standard" diet.

Over the past decade there has been a change in what is referred to as "standard" brought about by the health epidemic that has captured the attention of everyone *and* anyone with the slightest of interests in health *and* fitness. This epidemic is the result of what we have witnessed world-wide, *not* country-specific anymore, but what is affecting the lifestyle of the young, teenagers, young adults, the mature, and the more life-experienced.

Interestingly, those that are more "life-experienced" representative of the more mature generations, are in fact the ones who are not *as* affected due to the habits they developed in their younger years. But, as we track backwards to the mature and young adults – the generations who are conceiving and nurturing the young and teenagers of tomorrow, there are worrisome trends. These are the generations that *somewhere* along the line when processed foods became more readily available, put aside what they once knew – the importance of a *balanced* diet. As a direct consequence, health *and* fitness in these generations is no longer commonplace and thus the young and teenagers are *missing out* on what they need to know.

In order to stop this "missing out", *The Secrets to Optimal Wellbeing* is aimed at the young adult foremost, followed by those closest to this generation – the mature and the teenage, to begin to bring back this *balanced* diet. Yet, to bring back balance we first must *restore* and *teach* the body what nourishes us and what consumes us – starting with limiting processed foods and consuming more *natural* vitamins and minerals: fruits and vegetables.

By focusing a nutrition plan of "more" fruits and vegetables and "less" processed foods – which is inclusive of meat-based products, our gut is able to afresh. Through this renewal, our bodies are capable of becoming more aware of what gives us energy (food sources) and what detracts from this energy source. But we need to start with the "less" and the "more" to kick-start not only our metabolism's efficiency, but to know ourselves better. By knowing the balance between "less" and "more" firsthand, this affords us the opportunity to pass on these nutritious traits to those we are responsible for nurturing – the generations of tomorrow. No matter who you are or where you are from, tomorrow's generation is our responsibility, your responsibility – but first we need to start with our generation to ensure the generations of tomorrow are more aware of their personal *wellbeing*. It starts with you – all of you.

Featured Recipes:

Chicken & Coriander Salad
Fish Salad
Indian Infused Siru Curry
Jaw Dropping Chicken Burgers
Lightly Spiced Roast Chicken
Masala Infused Chicken Stirfry
Seasoned Chicken
Seasoned Fish
Spiced Chicken & Mushrooms
Spiced Chicken Spinach Wrap
Spinach & Salmon Salad

To follow, recipes in 2.5 *do* contain meat-based products and are easily and readily interchangeable. These have been kept to a minimum and form the basis for you – providing you with the "keys" to still have meat-based meals, but alongside your more dominant vegetable-based meals. Going forward, the 12 Week Guide is all about giving you *The Secrets to Optimal Wellbeing* and this is a significant contributor – "less" meat throughout the 12 Weeks whilst consuming "more" fruits and vegetables. There are *no* off-limit foods, but by refining the meals we consume using the *less versus more* cue, you will be one step closer to achieving your *optimal wellbeing*.

2.5.1 Chicken & Coriander Salad

Ingredients:
Chicken (100g)
Coriander (1/4 cup, chopped finely)
Mushrooms (1 ½ cups)
Wombok (1 ½ cups)
Ricotta (50g)
Cherry Tomatoes (100g)
Salt and Pepper (to taste)
Olive Oil

Preparation time:
30 minutes

Serves:
2

Nutrition friendly:
Gluten-Free

Guide:
Slice chicken breasts into manageable pieces, lightly coast with salt and pepper then place under grill being sure to turn until cooked through and tender.
Finely slice coriander and add to salad bowl.
Slice mushrooms and wombok– add to salad bowl.
Chop wombok lengthways and then into halves – add to salad bowl.
Slice cherry tomatoes into quarters – add to salad bowl.
Once the chicken has cooked through, add to salad bowl allowing the heat to lightly steam the mushrooms and wombok.
Using your fingers, lightly crumble the ricotta over the top of the salad with the salt and pepper (to taste), lightly mixing through the ingredients through the salad.
Done!
Tag your salad on Topicthread to be added to our gallery!

2.5.2 Fish Salad

Ingredients:

Fish (100g, of choice)
Tomato (1)
Mushrooms (1/2 cup)
Cabbage (1/2 cup)
Broccoli (1/2 cup)
Spiced Olives (20g)
Ginger (20g)
Minced garlic (1 teaspoon)
Minced ginger (1 teaspoon)
Chilli Flakes (1 tablespoon)
Olive Oil
Salt and Pepper (to season)

Preparation time:
20 minutes

Serves:
2

Nutrition friendly:
Gluten-Free

Guide:
Bring frying pan to heat and drizzle lightly with olive oil. Place fish into frying pan. Add chilli flakes, minced garlic and ginger to frying pan. Allow fish to cook through until ready then take off the heat.
Slice mushroom and cabbage finely and add to salad bowl.
Chop tomato into cubes and roughly chop broccoli into edible pieces.
Slice spiced olives and ginger finely – add to salad bowl.
Add fish to salad bowl and gently stir through ingredients adding salt and pepper to taste.
Done!

Tag your salad on Topicthread to be added to our gallery!

2.5.3 Indian Infused Siru Curry

Ingredients:
Chicken (500g)
Tomatoes (1 can, diced)
Masala (2 tablespoons)
Curcumin (2 tablespoons)
Chilli Flakes (1 tablespoon)
Natural Yoghurt (1/3 cup)
Crushed Garlic (2 tablespoons)
Crushed Ginger (2 tablespoons)
Salt (1 tablespoon)
Rice (2 cups)

Preparation time:
60 minutes

Serves:
6

Nutrition friendly:
Gluten-Free

Guide:

Slice chicken breasts into manageable pieces and put aside.

Heat saucepan and once brought to boil - add rice.

Bring saucepan to heat and add can of tomatoes and *all* spices. Let sauce simmer for 10-15 minutes.

Check on rice – once cooked through set aside to cool.

Add sliced chicken to sauce and simmer for a further 30 minutes.

Add yoghurt to desired consistency (if you would like less of a reduced sauce, you may choose to leave this).

Let simmer for a further 5 minutes ensuring checking the texture of the chicken – once it has reached desired tenderness take off the heat.

Add rice to serving bowls with desired amount of your now ready to serve Siru curry.

Done!

Tag your curry on Topicthread to be added to our gallery!

2.5.4 Jaw Dropping Chicken Burgers

Ingredients:
Burger:
Bread Roll (2, of choice)
Spinach (30g)
Tomato (1)
Mozzarella Cheese (30g)
Pineapple (30g)
Pickled Ginger (20g)
Mushroom (30g)
Aioli Sauce (to dress)
Chicken Patties:
Minced Chicken (200g)
Chilli Flakes (1 teaspoon)
Minced Garlic (1 teaspoon)
Minced Ginger (1 teaspoon)
Parsley (1 teaspoon)
Soy Sauce (1 tablespoon)
Olive Oil (to lightly fry)
Rice Breadcrumbs (enough to coat patties)

Preparation time:
30 minutes

Serves:
2

Nutrition friendly:
Open

Guide:
To make chicken patties add mince together with spices
along with the parsley, finely cut, into mixing bowl.
Once herbs have been stirred through, using your hands,
place patties into a bowl filled with the breadcrumbs and
lightly coat.

Once you have coated your patties, bring frying pan to heat with a drizzle of oil and cook until golden brown.

Open your bread rolls into halves, ready for the ingredients to be added.

Place spinach onto bread roll, followed by the tomato and mushrooms – evenly distributing ingredients onto the two bread rolls.

Add chicken patty onto bread roll followed by the mozzarella cheese to allow it to melt lightly over the hot patty.

Add the pineapple, then the ginger.

Lastly, add the aioli sauce onto the top half of the bread roll then close up.

Done!

Tag your chicken burger on Topicthread to be added to our gallery!

2.5.5 Lightly Spiced Roast Chicken

Ingredients:
Whole Small Chook (Chicken)
Thyme (1 tablespoon)
Garlic Salt (2 tablespoons)
Chilli Flakes (1 tablespoon)
Chilli Powder (1 tablespoon)
Olive Oil

Preparation time:
75 minutes

Serves:
4

Nutrition friendly:
Gluten-Free

Guide:
Preheat oven to 200C and prepare baking tray.
Season chicken with spices (thyme, garlic salt, chilli flakes and chilli powder) by rubbing gently into the skin.
Lightly drizzle with olive oil and then place into oven.
Option: to stuff chicken mix breadcrumbs with the spices (additional servings) and bring together with a pinch of olive oil.
Place chook into oven for 15 minutes on 200-210C then reduce to 170 for 25-30 minutes. Check to see density of chook thereafter and then leave on 150 for a further 15 minutes.
Let cool and then slice to serve.
Done!

Tag your roast chicken on Topicthread to be added to our gallery!

2.5.6 Masala Infused Chicken Stir-fry

Ingredients:
Chicken (100g)
Sundried Tomatoes (20g)
Mushrooms (50g)
Cucumber (1/4 cup)
Spinach (30g)
Masala (Spice, 1 Tablespoon)
Olive Oil
Cheese (handful to dress)

Preparation time:
20 minutes

Serves:
2

Nutrition friendly:
Gluten-Free

Guide:
Slice chicken (breasts) finely then add to heated pan adding a drizzle of olive oil.
Add mushrooms to pan, finely sliced.
Add sundried tomatoes to pan – lowering the heat.
Add masala to pan – sprinkle over pan ingredients and let simmer on low heat.
Pull a part spinach with your fingers – add to pan.
Slice cucumber into cubes then add to pan.
Stir through ingredients gently.
When ready to serve, add the cheese and gently stir through.
Done!

Tag your stir-fry on Topicthread to be added to our gallery!

2.5.7 Seasoned Chicken

Ingredients:
Chicken (100g)
Sundried Tomatoes (30g)
Mushrooms (50g)
Pepper (1 teaspoon)
Chilli Flakes (1 teaspoon)
Minced Garlic (1 teaspoon)
Olive Oil
Thyme (1 teaspoon)

Preparation time:
20 minutes

Serves:
2

Nutrition friendly:
Gluten-Free

Guide:
Slice chicken breasts finely and add to heated pan (or wok).
Add a drizzle of olive oil – adding mushrooms and the sliced sundried tomatoes to pan.
Stir through ingredients and then add spices: pepper, chilli flakes, minced garlic, and thyme.
Mix spices into the pan ingredients – simmer until chicken is cooked through and nice and tender.
Serve with your choice of mixed salad (optional).
Done!

Tag your chicken on Topicthread to be added to our gallery!

2.5.8 Seasoned Fish

Ingredients:
Fish (4 pieces, Basa)
Chilli Flakes (1 tablespoon)
Garlic (2 tablespoons)
Lemon Juice (1 tablespoon)
Pepper (1 teaspoon)
Olive oil

Preparation time:
20 minutes

Serves:
4

Nutrition friendly:
Gluten-Free

Guide:
Bring frying pan to heat and lightly drizzle bottom with oil.
Add fish pieces.
Evenly spread chilli flakes, garlic, pepper and lemon juice over all pieces of fish.
When cooked through, turn and coat fish pieces with sauce formed in the frying pan.
Let fish simmer until cooked through and fish pieces have soaked through with the sauce.
Serve with your choice of mixed salad.
Done!

Tag your fish on Topicthread to be added to our gallery!

2.5.9 Spiced Chicken & Mushrooms

Ingredients:
Chicken (400g)
Mushroom (200g)
Chilli Flakes (2 tablespoons)
Chilli Powder (1 tablespoon)
Pepper (1 tablespoon)
Salt (1 tablespoon)
Olive Oil

Preparation time:
30 minutes

Serves:
4

Nutrition friendly:
Gluten-Free

Guide:
Slice chicken (breasts) finely into strips then proceed to add to heated frying pan lightly drizzled with olive oil.
Slice mushrooms and add to frying pan.
Let mushrooms sizzle down to size and coat chicken with chilli flakes, chilli powder, pepper and salt – stirring through to blend with all chicken strips.
When chicken is almost done, remove the juices that have formed in the frying pan (being careful not to remove any pockets of flavour) – let chicken and mushrooms sizzle for a further 5 minutes before removing from the heat.
Serve with your choice of mixed salad (optional).
Done!

Tag your chicken & mushroom on Topicthread to be added to our gallery!

2.5.10 Spiced Chicken Spinach Wrap

Ingredients:
Chicken (100g)
Spinach (30g)
Mushrooms (50g)
Cheese (grated, 50g)
Tomatoes (1 can, diced)
Masala (1 teaspoon)
Curcumin (1 teaspoon)
Chilli Flakes (1 teaspoon)
Tomato Paste (1 tablespoon)
Olive Oil
Wraps (2, spinach infused suggested)

Preparation time:
30 minutes

Serves:
2

Nutrition friendly:
Gluten-Free

Guide:
Slice chicken breasts finely and add to heated saucepan lightly coated with olive oil. Add spices to saucepan then add can of tomatoes. Let simmer until the sauce slowly thickens.

Add tomato paste, if necessary, to reach the thickened consistency as desired.

Slice mushrooms finely. Lay down both wraps and coat with spinach followed by the sliced mushrooms.

Using a draining-scoop (to limit the amount of sauce onto the wrap) add chicken to the wrap. Add or limit sauce as desired (note: the more sauce you add the messier the wrap will become).

Lastly, add cheese on top of the heated chicken, allowing it to lightly melt, then proceed to tuck the bottom of the wrap upwards and then fold in the sides.
Done!

Tag your wrap on Topicthread to be added to our gallery!

2.5.11 Spinach & Salmon Salad

Ingredients:

Smoked Salmon (200g)   Spinach (1/2 cup)
Ricotta (50g)   Stuffed Olives (20g)
Tomatoes (2)   Cucumber (1/4 cup)
Purple Cabbage (1/2   Capsicum (1/2)
cup)

Preparation time:
20 minutes

Serves:
2

Nutrition friendly:
Gluten-Free

Guide:
Slice tomatoes into cubes and then squeeze lightly to drain excess juices before adding to salad bowl.
Chop the spinach and cabbage finely, rinse under cold water then add to salad bowl.
Chop cucumber into cubes then add to salad bowl.
Slice capsicum into cubes being sure to remove all seeds, then add to salad bowl.
Chop olives into quarters then add to salad bowl.
Finely pull a part the smoked salmon into strips and add to salad bowl.
Lastly, using your fingers lightly crumble the ricotta on top of the salad bowl. Once the ricotta is all crumbled, use your fingers to gently mix the ingredients together being careful not to scrunch the salmon.
Done!

Tag your salad on Topicthread to be added to our gallery!

Closing thoughts

Your metabolism will thank you. Your exterior appearance will begin to shine brighter than before. You are essentially restoring the *good* vitamins and minerals back into your skin through increasing their presence in your daily nutrition. Internally, your body will thank you – progressively restoring it towards its point of *optimal wellbeing*. And your "vibes" will begin to transition towards a healthier outlook that in turn acts as a catalyst towards the *want* to hold onto this new and renewed lifestyle.

Initially, Part 2 presented section 2.1 that outlined the ease and simplicity of following a vegan, raw *and* gluten-free nutrition plan. But, committing to a raw nutrition plan isn't for everyone and this has always been understood – the premise behind providing a sample of recipes. By providing a select portion of recipes, these provide you with the tools to choose whether or not you choose to eat raw – stimulating your digestive system, within limitations, whilst consuming *all* the vitamins and minerals the fruit and/or vegetable has to offer.

A result of cooking fruits and/or vegetables is that we can lose a "chunk" of their vitamins and minerals on offer. Cooking essentially further breaks down the food source for us, in contrast to our bodies digesting the food as a whole. However, by cooking our fruits and/or vegetables it is important to note that we are *not* at a substantial loss – the importance is on consuming these types of energy sources. By sporadically consuming raw meals and including these in our diet from time, our metabolism is kept on its toes – contributing to its efficiency in breaking down (digesting) our energy sources. Raw foods are a good thing – *not* a bad thing, but does *not* have to always be applied, rather form the basis and foundations of this Guide.

These foundations thus featured throughout section 2.2 where vegetarian recipes were presented alongside primarily gluten-free *and* vegan meals. Although raw ingredients were featured in a significant number of recipes, primarily the majority of meals were *not* entirely raw, providing a variety of options for you to *choose* – vegetarian, vegan, raw and/or gluten-free, not just one.

The meals we consume in between our primarily meals – snacks, were then discussed and presented in sections 2.3 (muffins) and 2.4 (smoothies). The recipes featured were not only vegetarian, *but* the majority of muffins were and can be easily made gluten-free by substituting the type of flour used. The same applies for vegan – *removing* the dairy can and is an option to be remembered and will not disrupt the overall recipe in the majority of cases i.e. cow milk to soy milk or the removal of eggs completely. Section 2.4 is *entirely raw* with all recipes comprising of a variety of fruits that are then blended. Bananas were heavily featured due to their smooth texture when blended and its ability to bind together other fruits whilst keeping an even blend.

Meat-based meals were then discussed in 2.5 with a selection of recipes provided. These recipes form the backbone for meat inclusive recipes. A sample of meals were presented and how they can be incorporated into your weekly nutrition Guide. Being mindful of the *objective*: gut health and restoration leading towards your *optimal wellbeing*, is key to keeping your gut health on track towards its restored state. Meat-based meals therefore have been incorporated into your 12 Week Guide, yet kept to a minimum for one reason: to allow your digestive system to regain control of how your body metabolises its food, working with *you* hereon in to achieve your *optimal wellbeing*.

The nutrition component of the Guide has now been discussed and you will find its 12 Week layout in Part 4 – but before that, Part 3 is now to come. In order to learn *The Secrets to Optimal Wellbeing*, your fitness is a key factor. It is important, however, when following a *fitness* Guide, that it is functional – allowing you to train your body most optimally and efficiently. Thus, the time has now come to take the reins of your new and renewed lifestyle by learning the "ropes" of the part-in-parcel of the Guide – your fitness, and how to apply functional movements to get the most out of the time spent towards developing your healthier *and* fitter lifestyle.

PART 3

FUNCTIONAL MOVEMENT

FITNESS

Outline

T he essence of functional movement is to provide the back-bone of *all* effective and lifestyle based training programs. By applying functional movement *patterns* you are learning and conditioning your body to use "movements" for *life* that will *not* lead to the onset nor cause injury. Functional movement, in itself, is a banner term for *movements* that are *functional* – whereby the human body moves how it was designed to move in contrast to moving in an unnatural state and thus placing increased loads on parts of the body that were *not* designed to withstand these loads.

The objective of Part 3 is to provide you with the keys to *optimal wellbeing* – laying out the "how to" when performing your "exercises" – at home *or* wherever you choose to take them. The exercises set out in Part 4 are primarily touched on herein, in one way, shape or form – giving you *not* the answers, but key technical parameters to follow and adhere to throughout employing the Guide.

Through performing exercises that are identified as functional movements, this allows you to "condition" more than one muscle at a time. For example, by effectively performing a *standard* squat whilst applying functional movement parameters, you are able to work (strengthen and condition) your (1) quadriceps, (2) hamstrings, (3) gluteus maximus, (4) dual calf muscle, (5) core, (6) lower back and a variety of (7) foot muscles – all in the *one* functional exercise.

To ensure the *fitness* Guide herein is streamlined, exercises that you will learn and perform over the 12 Weeks are segmented into "body" sections. These sections are of primary focus due to body design – whereby our bodies are designed to work interchangeably with various muscle-groups. By applying functional movement patterns and parameters, we are able to work "more" muscle-groups in the "one" exercise. This form of collaborative exercise is centred on the body's design and thus synced with our natural state. These exercises replicate "movements" that are more often than not performed in our daily lives. And as a result of working *more than* one muscle at a time – functional movements allow the presented Guide to be simplified *and* time efficient.

The "how to" will now be discussed and act as a point of reference throughout your 12 Week Plan and onwards. Part 3 will now discuss your *form* and *technique* when applying these at-home centred exercises, starting with 3.1 – back, then 3.2 – chest, followed by 3.3 – legs, before 3.4 – core, and lastly 3.5 – aerobic, where the cardio components of your *fitness* Guide is featured. And remember, this is your *choice*, towards your renewed lifestyle – you've got the reins in both hands and Part 3 is one step closer towards a healthier *and* fitter you!

3.1 Back

Before commencing any movement sequence, there are two key techniques to remember, always. These techniques contribute towards applying effective functional movements and will be reiterated at the beginning of each section for good measure – they are your *form* Guide.

Technique 101 – Shoulders back and down: to achieve this position, draw your shoulders back then slightly lift them towards your neck in a mini "shrug-back" and then drop them down. You will "feel" this by your shoulder blades being "tucked-in" – *think*, your wings are secured.

Technique 101 – Belly-button towards your spine: to achieve this position, if standing up – stand nice and tall, if sitting down, sit nice and tall, and if laying down, lay nice and long (tall). Now, the idea here is to "tighten" your core – activating your muscles, preparing them for use! Likened to flexing your abdominal muscles, whether you can see them *or* not, focus on drawing back your belly-button towards your spine. You aren't "sucking in" your stomach, but rather tightening. Once you have achieved this position your stomach will feel firmer to you, and isn't necessarily felt by all externally, but internally, this sensation shall appear.

Now let's begin:

When working out your back, you will find one primary technique used throughout the Guide – the *pulling* movement. By performing a pulling movement, you are drawing on your back muscles – activating them and in turn, conditioning them through applying load. In order to perform pulling exercises most effectively, your shoulders need to be "back and down" and your belly-button "drawn" towards your spine.

In your home environment, you are able to strengthen your back by following simply steps discussed in the Guide. For example, when asked to find a **skipping rope**, it is important that it is a sturdy rope that can hold your own weight i.e. will not snap under pressure. You will be asked to "hook" this piece of rope around objects that *can* hold your pulling weight – you pulling the rope *without* the item moving. Or, you pulling the rope whilst the item *progressively* moves, slowly.

Objects that aren't easily "moveable" include: the tire on your car, a heavy-set couch, or a solid-wood office desk, for example. Objects to be considered when using a longer rope, due to their potential to "move" towards you, include: a washing machine, large stones and/or bricks, or a bedframe, for example. When the time comes to *roll* or *push* an object, consider items that you can move – but *not* with ease. These are to be lower set objects and may include: a tire, a table, or a couch, for example. These are all merely examples, but it is important to take **caution** when thinking of "tall" objects – these are to be steered clear of as there is potential for them to fall towards you. Please do *not* take this risk. Be smart and choose objects that are at a lower height and can be *pulled*.

You will be asked to pull either the object – *or* yourself. If you are pulling an object, remember to maintain *form* and to pull the object one pull at a time towards you. The objective is *not* to get the object to you, but to use the object as a *load* that is being "pulled" by your **back** – conditioning *and* strengthening your back muscles all the whilst working your core.

Whether you are standing or sitting – technique is important. When standing, maintain a tall posture whilst keeping your shoulders back and down, and your belly-button drawn towards your spine. If you are required to be seated (on the floor), keep your legs in front of you with a slight bend at the knees –

keeping the soles of your feet off the ground, *activating* your core with each and every pulling motion.

Being mindful of "what" your body is doing when performing pulling movements will bring awareness to how your body moves and how it responds when under pressure *or* load. When pulling, ensure *both* hands hold the rope and/or object firmly, *but* in a manner that is comfortable. Keep both hands *sideways* whilst gripped, pulling your hands back towards your sides – stopping when your elbows *pass* your back. There is no need to go beyond this point due to the potential strain then placed on your shoulders and thus being *no longer* functional.

To get the most out of your back exercises, closely follow the Guide and remember your *technique* and *form*. Meanwhile, to displace the age-old myth of "will strength training make me bigger" – in short: no, but it will make you firmer, tighter, *and* stronger. Depending on your **genetic build**, which is unique to us all, some of us more easily gain muscle *whilst others* take a little longer. If you do have a more muscle-prone build, the good news is that this comes *hand-in-hand* with a more efficient metabolism. Yet, if you don't acquire muscle as easily, your strength work can be seen as "aerobic" work which in turn then contributes to a healthier *and* fitter you – it's up to your genetic build. As for the **scale** – *look away*. A well-known *fact* is that muscle weighs *three times* more than fat, thus your numbers will go *up* initially, then decline as your body becomes more **balanced**.

3.2 Chest

When it comes to performing the chest-specific exercises throughout the Guide, it is important to "lock and load" – accomplished by following Technique 101 principles.

Technique 101 – shoulders back and down (see 3.1) & belly-button towards your spine (see 3.1)

To optimise the functionality of your upper body, your back (3.1) goes hand-in-hand with your chest. It is common for these two muscle-group to not be given their fair share, with the chest often being given the spotlight. But, if the back is not conditioned to the same degree as the back, this is where muscle imbalances will appear and develop, compromising your *optimal wellbeing*. In order to keep on the "straight and narrow" and avoid imbalances, the chest is to be given the same attention as the back, and vice versa.

By working our back and chest in unison, following a balanced program, our upper bodies become not only stronger, but more functional in our day to day lives. And to dispel the myth of "will my chest get smaller" the simple answer is: muscle progressively overrides fat, thus the fat becomes "firmer" and the muscle contributes to your overall muscle mass, speeding up the efficiency of your metabolism! It all works together.

When it comes to strengthening and conditioning your chest, there are a multitude of at-home based exercises that can help. The Guide presented in Part 4 will explain "what" to perform, but herein offers additional information to the "how" during the course of your Guide. It is important to follow the Guide and refer to Part 3 consistently whilst being mindful of the parameters set throughout – helping shape your awareness and application how to employ functional movement patterns.

You will be prompted to find a table, at times – this is to be around hip height to allow enough of a "fall" but not too deep, unless specified. Most commonly, you will be doing what is known as a "push-up" but in modified versions. Against a table, your feet will be behind – pretend you are leaning against the table with your hands shoulder width a part and your backside flat; endeavour to keep a straight line so that your backside is not disrupting the shape of your line i.e. straight back. To perform the push action, you will be asked to lower your chest towards the edge of the table – it is not necessary to "touch" the edge, but until your elbows reach a 90-degree angle – then proceed to push yourself back up.

There's more. A modified version of the push-up will include lowering yourself to the floor in the push-up position, yet instead of being on your toes you will be on your knees all the whilst being mindful of a straight back and keeping your backside *tucked* opposed to out. A progression of this version is to place one arm out straight – leaving you with *one* arm to perform the push-up. This is a challenging movement, however ensuring you're following **technique 101** parameters, you will be able to draw on your core to perform this move all the whilst strengthening your stabilizers.

Using around the home "bottles" will be necessary. Examples include: milk bottles, soft-drink bottles, or juice bottles Essentially, these bottles will act as *free weights* and the only prerequisite is to ensure you can hold onto them comfortably. To perform a chest press with these bottles, it is necessary to stand tall and to start with both bottles against your side. From here you will lift the bottles to shoulder height and then proceed to *push* outwards – away from you, until your arms have straightened. When pushing your arms outwards, aim for both bottles to meet, creating a triangle with your body. To lower, bring the bottles back to your shoulders and then by your sides. To hold, keep the bottles raised at shoulder height, with elbows bent by your side – this is an *isometric hold* placing an enduring load on your muscles, increasing their ability to be maintained under pressure.

At times you will be asked to focus on one arm over the other – this is a form of isometric holds, before increasing the load all together. This means that instead of removing one of your hands from "holding" the weight, you will be asked to push through one arm opposed to the other, and vice versa. This begins to prepare your body for withstanding increased loads in contrast to "jumping" straight to it. Performing exercises that you have "jumped" to and *not* progressed towards limits the functionality of the exercises due to your muscles being compromised under pressure. Therefore, the Guide is set in place to build you towards these movements to ensure you stay on track towards *optimal wellbeing*.

At times you will be asked to focus on power. When performing exercises with power, this requires you to pull (3.1) or push (3.2) with force. For example, when standing close to a wall, pushing against the wall to propel yourself backwards – whilst maintaining a balanced state, works not only on your ability to develop and call on power, but your overall balance and thus body stabilizers.

Being mindful of these form and technique parameters will allow you to effectively *and* functionally perform the exercises presented in the Guide. By conditioning the chest, your posture will become taller – ensuring it is done *in sync* with your back. The common "slouch" many carry from conditioning their chest whilst neglecting the back, will be removed when *balancing* the two. The benefits of strengthening your upper body in unison contributes towards your overall functionality and ultimate daily movements.

3.3 Legs

With the technical parameters of the upper body discussed, it is time to zero-in on the lower body. Comprising of the largest muscle in our body, the lower body and its functionality is key to our movements in our day to day lives. By applying the principles of functional movement, you are able to work near *all* muscle-groups, in one form or another, when performing most exercises centred on conditioning the lower body – specifically your legs.

Being mindful of technique 101 principles (see 3.1), you are able to work "more of" your body through leg-based muscle-grouped exercises, over *any* other muscle-group. These exercises have the capacity to be modified into full-body exercises, at times, whereby you also "work" muscle-groups of your upper body. It can be done, and will be throughout the Guide in Part 4 and as a result herein, lower body form *and* technique indicators will be discussed.

Sitting down on a chair is pretty straight forward – right? What about sitting, but hovering – your backside is not allowed to touch the seat? This is a simple progression you will be asked to perform over the course of the Guide. But, "how" to sit *or* hover is key. The number one rule for all lower body exercises is:

your knees are to stay in front of your toes – never over

By ensuring your knees do *not* go beyond your toes when lowering yourself *or* bending ensures that your movements remain functional. The benefits of performing a functional movement is that it contributes towards your *optimal wellbeing* – it does *not* detract. Therefore, when asked to "sit" onto a chair, ensure you are standing tall with feet shoulder width a part – then bend your hips backwards, "poking" your backside outwards, then "dropping" down slowly towards the chair. It is important here to also remember **technique 101** parameters – shoulders back and down, *and* belly-button drawn towards your spine.

Progressions of this *squat* movement will call for you to "sit" against a wall. This requires you to keep a straight back and position yourself against a wall – then to lower yourself into the seated position all the whilst pressing your back slightly against the wall for support. This movement is all about your lower body whilst your upper body is being used as a support act. It is important when leaning against walls to ensure your lower body maintains **technique 101** parameters and that a 90-degree angle is created behind the back of your knees – your lowest height. If you're not quite able to "drop" down to reach this angle – this is okay; over the course of the Guide, this will come.

"How low you can go" is not the objective when conditioning your lower body. Movements are to be controlled and performed on a *one-count* opposed to being "over and done with". In order to perform functional movements, control is the objective. Thus, when asked to raise your leg when seated against the wall, this is to be counted on a *one-count*: one-count, two-count, three-count – and then held for **one**-count before being lowered to the same count, back to the floor.

Other than the squat movement, you will also be asked to lunge throughout the course of the Guide. To perform a lunge, functionally, keeping your knees in front of your toes is rule number one. Then, technique 101 parameters. Now you are ready. Standing upright, take a step back with one leg and allow your knee then to touch the ground. Check your *form* – are your *wings* locked in and is your core *activated*? Ensuring your form is set, lift your knee slightly off the ground. By now you would have noticed your front leg *will be bent* too, after all, as we can't place one knee on the ground without bending the other, whilst applying bodily control.

To perform the "lunge" keep your feet exactly where they are, then begin to straighten your back leg whilst keeping your front leg slightly bent. The *down* movement – one leg steps back, almost touches the ground, holds – then the up movement – progresses to the "standing tall" position. The *lunge* comes in two sequences – repetitive *or* interchanging. If repetitive, this is where you'll be asked to focus on the one leg and repeat the lunge movement before changing to the opposite leg. If interchanging, this is where you'll be asked to perform one lunge on "leg A" then one lunge on "leg B" and repeat until your set has been completed. In between each lunge it is important to stand tall and check your **technique 101** parameters whilst keeping an eye out for your knees and that they *are not* too close to your toes.

Now that you know the "how" behind the lunge, the "how" behind the *free-squat* can be highlighted. Likened to the example provided about wall *and* chair squats, the free-squat requires you to sit "anywhere" but without *any* support. To balance, place your arms out in front of you and then "poke" your backside out – then drop down, keeping a straight back and allowing your *natural arch* to remain. You will notice your heels will begin to "dig" into the ground to maintain a sturdy base of support – this is good! And by keeping tabs on your form *and* technique will allow you to not only *control* your movements, but ensure that they are consistently functional.

Lower body progressions call on the use of power. To perform power movements it is important to first check your form and technique. Once you are satisfied that you have achieved a functional position, you will generate force through the ground to propel yourself into the air – in two ways. One, when squatting to propel yourself into the air, lower yourself to the 90-degree angle stance (required behind your knees), then push through your soles to lift off – ever so slightly. You will then be asked to regain and/or maintain this position and repeat. Two, when lunging to propel yourself into the air, once your back leg is lowered you are going to "come up" and switch to the next leg – in the *air*. To do this you need to push through your soles to quickly transition between the two.

In order to "walk through" *air-jumps*, stand tall and switch your legs back and forth – pretending your feet are on opposite sides of a line, switching them on opposing sides of this "line" before proceeding to add a *bend* in your knees. This form also replicates the initial progression of "toe taps" which comes *prior* to lifting off into the *air* – in a refined stance rather than the widened lunge extension. Once you have practiced this walk through, it is time to *air-jump* – do this nice and slow. It is important to remember that it doesn't matter if you make it high *or* low, it's all about you – your progressions, your development, and your capacity to maintain balance: it is *all* individual, it is all about you.

It is key to remember when it comes to your lower body, your upper body plays a part in maintaining your balance, contributing to your ultimate movement and its functionality. By conditioning our upper body, it affords us *more* control of our lower body – but if we neglect this, our bodies become unbalanced. The same is said for our lower body – if equal emphasis isn't placed on these muscle-groups our all-round functionality isn't as efficient and hinders our bodily control. In order to tie these two together, our upper and lower muscle-groups, the *core* holds the **key** and "why" it forms one of the reinforced technical parameters.

3.4 Core

Applying functional movement parameters to strength and conditioning *actives*, allows us to work more than one muscle-group at a time, affording time efficiency and the inclusion of exercises that are working *with* our bodies design, not against. For example, when we twist our bodies – specifically our muscles, we are compromising not only the effectiveness of the exercise, but we are increasing the load on our body whilst under *strain* – completely different to applying pressure. When our muscles are strained, think knotted – they can get caught and ultimately conditioned to function in this way. As a result, functional movement goes out the door and our bodily control is compromised.

A key muscle-group that acts as a "monitor" of sorts for functional movements, is our core. By ensuring **technique 101** parameters are followed, specifically ensuring your belly-button is *drawn* towards your spine, "locks in" your body's centre, calling on its adjoining muscle-groups. As a result, this locked-in behaviour allows us to work more than one muscle-group at a time. However, if our core falls by the wayside, this becomes more difficult and is why progressively conditioning our core to *activate* is emphasised and thus a part of the Guide provided in Part 4.

By implementing the Guide in Part 4 you will steadily learn to condition your core. In order to *functionally* do this, gone are the days of the "sit-up" – it is not functional. Why? Because not only does it strain your neck muscles, if you're yet to develop and acquire a certain level of strength, you're unable to efficiently and effectively call on the muscles needed to perform this movement. This is why so many have tried the sit-up and often given up due to its contribution to discomfort and lack of bodily control. You might ask, should I ignore this exercise all together? Not necessarily. Yet, it is not a functional movement. The sit-up is an isometric exercise targeting your core – but unless you would prefer to spend more time working your core in contrast to less, then – go for it. This movement nonetheless is excluded from the Guide due to its lack of functionality.

Included in the Guide are a variety of ways to condition your core, functionally. For example, there will be times when you will be asked to lay down on the floor. From here it is important to remember your now familiar **technique 101** parameters and then proceed with your back flat on the floor – removing your arch. To do this, you may feel like you are "curving" your spine – this is okay providing you are laying "tall" and that your body is straight; your heels are touching the ground and so too is the back of your head. From here there are various movements you will perform.

Whilst laying on the floor, ensuring your form *and* technique follows the core guidelines, you will be asked to point your toes straight and to keep your arms by your side. One progression from here is to lift your toes off the ground so that your feet are hovering in the air – the lower the *lift-hold* the more difficult. This movement has multiple options. You will lift to a *one-count* and then lower, the height is at your discretion – remembering to work with your individual level of fitness. To progress, keep your palms upwards, *not* allowing help from your arms. Once you have lifted your feet *off* the ground, ensure your back stays *flat* and that your arch does not reappear – we want to keep our *form*.

Furthermore, whilst laying on the floor another functional core movement will ask you to maintain your straight back – *arch-free*, then proceed to lift your knees towards your chest, keeping a 90-degree angle behind both knees. From this position you need to "think" you are riding a bicycle. One leg will begin to almost straighten, toes pointed, and then you will tuck it back towards your core whilst your other leg begins to "cycle" and create its own circle. Remember to be mindful of your *technique* whilst riding!

A refined movement in the cycle position is all about *control*. You will be asked to bring your knees to your chest, but from here, whilst being mindful of your *technique*, you are to straighten them, slowly, lowering them back to the ground. It will be noticeable that the slower you go, the more you're conditioning your core – a *progression*.

Another progression will call on you to remain on the floor, being mindful of your form and technique. When you're set, lift your feet slightly off the ground, enough to *air-kick* with *both* legs. Think: *scissor-kick* – you will be controlling your legs whilst they kick up and down, all the whilst holding onto your form *and* technique. This movement is done in *one-counts* – this means you will need to scissor-kick for a period of time before you can lower your feet back to the ground.

Rather than laying on your back, there will be times where you'll need to roll over *onto* your stomach. But you won't stay there for long. From this position, you need to raise your body onto your *toes* and *elbows* – your lower body will be raised and your upper body weighted through your elbows. Your core is the one here that is to *hold it* all together. Having taken away all of your support, this is one movement that forces you to *activate* your core. However, if your form *or* technique flails, your lower back will weaken. Therefore, it is important to ensure your back is *straight*, your backside is tucked in, and that your arch is primarily removed – allowing you to concentrate on activating your core, and *holding* it. Known as the **plank**, it is an isometric exercise that is beneficial to conditioning the core and its endurance.

Once you have learned to control *and* activate your core, there are a variety of exercises you can perform that will in fact condition your core simply by you *choosing* to activate it. This includes *even* walking. One exercise that draws on the stability of your core, whilst helping you *develop* control is a "slow-twist" from side to side. To perform this movement, you will need "bottles" mentioned in 3.2 – an object you can hold onto comfortably with *both* hands, yet *heavy* enough that you wouldn't want to keep holding it for *too* long. Being mindful of your form *and* technique, hold the object out in front of you, creating a 90-degree angle at both elbows. Your arms will be bent. From here, rotate to your left, keeping your core in position whilst turning – until the object has moved to be *parallel* with your side. Then "from here", turn slowly back to your centre and then proceed to twist to your right – no further than your side, ensures the "slow-twist" remains functional.

The core forms the "action centre" of all functional movements. By progressively working towards controlling your core and activating it, your bodily control will improve and continuously progress. In addition, your ability to efficiently perform and execute functional movements will become commonplace and in turn your core will become a natural stabiliser. As this stabilisation is achieved, by activating your core without too much thought, your ability *and* efficiency to move functionally will develop, contributing towards your *optimal wellbeing*.

3.5 Aerobic

The featured Guide in Part 4 has two components: nutrition *and* fitness. With nutrition discussed in detail throughout Part 2, and up until now, Part 3 has discussed in depth performance parameters for fitness: strength and conditioning. Yet to be discussed is the aerobic component of this conditioning – the physicality incorporated in the Guide, which caps off the discussion of your overall fitness.

The role of the Guide ties nutrition *and* fitness together for one primary reason – often overlooked in any fad diet and neglected from lifestyle changes. The role that nutrition plays is that it affords you energy, whilst the role fitness plays is that is consumes it – the energy. It's straight forward. In order to maintain your *optimal wellbeing*, we need to find a balance between the two: nutrition and fitness. By finding a balance it allows us to play one off the other. The more we partake in fitness, essentially, the more fuel (food) our bodies need to use as energy.

The type of energy is one thing – and the restorative kind has been detailed in Part 2. But when it comes to fitness, there are countless activities you can partake in – some requiring more energy than others. Thus, with the objective of this Guide cantered on young adults and for its incorporation and consideration of and for *all* from the ground up, activities of focus are *not* centred on performance, yet work towards your *optimal wellbeing*. By all means, once you have taken the reins of your renewed lifestyle, this is where and when you will be physically capable, and able, to take on board any activity of choice that adds to your happiness – you'll have the bodily control to do so!

Keeping the objective of the Guide in mind, the aerobic component is designed for "non-elites" – you aren't quite sure how to get started, you might know but somewhere along the way you hit a road bump, *or* you know but at times it gets tricky to put into action what you know – *or*, you've read and heard of that many, and that much conflicting information, the time has come to create and put into place a lifestyle that is suited for *you* – as an individual, contributing towards your *optimal wellbeing*.

Starting from the ground up and being mindful that you need to crawl before you can walk, the aerobic proponent of Part 4 is all about walking and progressing towards getting a little bit quicker, and a little bit faster. But why walking? Essentially, walking can be progressed simply – from walk – to jog – then run – before sprint. Walking in itself is a functional movement *and* is one of the best beginning *catalysts* – it too is a lifestyle: whether you choose to walk, jog, run *or* sprint.

It isn't just about the walking, or the running. You will need a tennis ball or a *ball* that can bounce, is easily carried in one hand, and that you can move with and hold onto without tiring. This *ball* will be, and is used as a "tool" throughout the Guide to provide mental awareness and conditioning, to help you monitor your performance progressions, and is "a" *catalyst* behind the Guide: your *reason* is within and it is to be held through every step of your 12 Week Journey.

The Guide will ask you to frequently bounce and catch your ball, in intervals *or* by a time pattern. On other occasions, you will be asked to simply hold onto your ball for *purpose*. Throughout the Guide you will progress from a walk to a jog. It is important that you are mindful that the Guide is designed for you – for you to go at your own pace, at your own level, and to walk, jog, run or sprint to *your own* beat. When the Guide prompts you to go a little bit faster – this is your "fast" – when you're prompted to sprint, this is your "sprint" – time is only a measure of *duration*, it is not a measure of your performance other than being indicative of yours, and yours alone, performance progressions.

Minutes and seconds will be given for the duration you are to allocate to your aerobic fitness. On average, your aerobic fitness will be a commitment of 4-5 times per week for 30 minutes – that's all! With this in mind, the 30 minutes allocated are filled with *purpose* – the objective to lead you towards a healthier and fitter you, contributing towards your *optimal wellbeing*.

Whilst performing all aerobic activities, it is important to be mindful of **technique 101** parameters and your **heart rate**. It is advised to consult your local **physician** prior to commencing the Guide to receive the "green light" that you are set to take on a health and fitness program. The majority of us *are* "okay" yet some of "us" may need to take a *little* more caution due to pre-existing health conditions. Remember: it *is* better to be *safe* than sorry.

If you do have a pre-existing health condition, no problem. The Guide is yours – you're to work at *your* pace, within *your* limits, and towards *your* lifestyle that you want – you're given the tools to *make the choices*. It is important to get the nod from your physician to ensure your health is monitored – this is important for all, irrespective of a pre-existing condition or not. Again: it *is* better to be *safe* than sorry. The best part? Having your heart rate tracked will allow you to see its progressive improvements alongside your overall health! It's a **win-win**.

When it comes to equipment, besides the ball, the only other piece of equipment you will need that mightn't be found around the house – is a skateboard! Not only will this "toy" allow you to work on your balance, it allows you to dynamically condition one leg at a time, contributing towards your overall *strength* of balance. In turn, this kind of balance – dynamic, contributes towards your ultimate strength gains and thus the efficiency of your metabolism. The skateboard is also a "tool" to be used to perform toe taps – executed on a raised platform, providing *more for less*, whilst working our body as a *whole*.

The aerobic component of the Guide will provide you with the "what" and "how" to get one step closer towards a healthier *and* fitter you. All walking, jogging, running and/or sprinting is suggested outdoors. You will need a circuit to walk/jog/run/sprint on, and approximately a 100m stretch to jog/sprint, and at times, skate. The Guide will lead the way – all you need to do is *listen* to your body, *listen* to your physician, and ultimately *listen* to the Guide to take the reins and discover your *optimal wellbeing*.

Closing thoughts

The design of our bodies is *key* to consider when undertaking and performing *fitness* exercises and *movements*. By considering and applying functional movement parameters in your fitness Guide, this affords efficiency in conditioning more than one muscle-group at a time, whilst also providing you with insurance – longevity to move with minimal risk of injury.

The categorisation of your body and its muscle-groups, from yours back (3.1), chest (3.2), legs (3.3), and core (3.4), is key to recognise throughout your fitness endeavours. By being aware of these "groups" you are given control – you have the capacity to take the reins and *understand* your body and how it works.

The one aspect of *functional movement fitness* scarcely considered, is how it is applicable to your aerobic (3.5) conditioning. The key here is form *and* technique – it can be applied and maintained. The **technique 101** parameters – shoulders back and down, and to ensure your belly-button is drawn towards your spine, affords consistency in posture and thus reduces the onset of "slouch" or muscle "stiffness" due to putting measures (parameters) in place to control your body's posture, and control. The more advanced your conditioning becomes, the more you will find postural considerations are required as a result of the increased load placed on your body.

The fitness parameters outlined in Part 3 serve to create a stronger *and* fitter you – acting as a point of reference throughout your 12 Week Journey. Being mindful of your form *and* technique is key, whilst being aware of your *reason* is central to keeping a hold of the reins and executing your Guide as planned. Holding onto your "ball" throughout, specifically when executing the Guide's fitness component, is your reminder – reminding you constantly of *why* you started and *why* you *will* **finish**.

The upcoming Guide in Part 4 is designed specifically for you – the *young adult* wanting to take the reins of their health *and* fitness – acting as a catalyst to get you on track to the lifestyle you desire. For the more "advanced" yet *non-elites*, this Guide acts as a building block – to be tweaked and moulded towards *your* health and fitness wants and needs. To the *inaugural* young adult, this Guide has been created for you – the road map outlined in Part 1 comes apparent in Part 4, and is just that: your *road map* to your renewed lifestyle and your *choice* of choosing happiness.

It is now time to hand you over to Part 4 and begin your 12 Week Journey. *No matter* where you are around the world, *no matter* where your home is, *no matter* its size, *no matter* your size, *no matter* your level of fitness, *no matter* your present nutrition, *no matter* what has been. What *does matter* is what's to come, and that time to *matter* is now! Let's do this together. May I present to you: Par 4 – Your 12 Week Journey.

PART 4

YOUR 12 WEEK JOURNEY

Outline

Herein lies your Guide that will take you on your own health *and* fitness journey over the next 12 Weeks. It has been designed with the young adult in mind alongside those of you that have been looking for that elusive Guide that not only is fitness affirmative, but also nutritiously informative – they work together – in the **one** Guide. Simply, the Guide comprises of recipes that will work with you to restore and rejuvenate your gut, all the whilst working with your metabolism, giving your body back the "tools" it once had or has forgotten. It's about re-learning these tools and making them work with you. This means you have the reins – you're in control.

The nutrition component of the Guide is centred around two of your three primary meals: lunch and dinner, and three of your secondary meals in the form of snacks. One of your primary meals, breakfast, is not given to allow you to choose – to decide what is best. Breakfast can come in many forms, from a mix of breads or fruits, depending on your dietary needs (i.e. gluten-free or raw), through to a combination of carbohydrates, fats and proteins in one – at your fingertips in *snacks* (2.3). The choice is yours. It is all about you – whether that be vegetarian, vegan, raw *or* gluten-free, or a combination i.e. lactose intolerant. The recipes are there for you, they are set out – for you, but it is up to you to *choose* what your breakfast will comprise of, and what your meals are for the weekend. That's right – your weekends are on you.

Don't worry – your weekends are set aside for you to implement what you are learning. Remember, this is a lifestyle improvement and in order for it to be maintained and to become a part of the "rejuvenated" you, your weekends are when you'll be putting your newfound knowledge to the test – apply it, challenge yourself, create, make a mess, do whatever you *choose* so long as it's working *with* you and contributing towards your happiness.

The fitness component of the Guide sets you off at *three* strength sessions per week and *four* aerobic. Over time these will progress to four and five, respectively. At initial glance it may appear "full" but in retrospect what we are doing is creating a *habit* – consistency in and for your "new" lifestyle. In order to rejuvenate yourself, there needs to be a bit of stepping outside of your comfort zone – the objective of this Guide. But, the Guide is here to hold-your-hand – it will not let you wonder, it will not lead you astray, nor misguide you. But it will give you freedom, it will give you flexibility, it will give you control – but most of all, responsibility.

The time has come to take responsibility back for who you are and who you are becoming. And given that you are reading this, I am incredibly excited for the *who* you are becoming – I hope you're smiling just as wide as I am, for you! Over the upcoming weeks, you will begin to feel different – at first, a little tired from your increased activity but this is negated by your nutrition – so, it is important to use the Guide as a whole. It works both ways – you'll be eating different foods, some you're really not familiar with, so you will yearn for certain food sources you've become accustomed towards. This is where your willpower comes in – and your *reason*. By ensuring your fitness is maintained, progressively this will override these yearnings – you will find yourself wanting more of the *good*, and less of the *bad*, simply because food is energy and as your body becomes more efficient and demanding of energy, it wants the "good stuff" – patience.

The Guide is designed with your weekly fitness Guide in two parts: strength and aerobic, followed by your nutrition Guide. At times your fitness Guide will bring together your strength and aerobic sessions in one, whilst your nutrition Guide will remain consistent throughout. However, your nutrition Guide affords you flexibility for breakfasts and weekend meals, whilst your fitness Guide hands you the reins to choose times with daily allocations given (albeit tangible).

In order to track-down the recipes for each individual meal – the Contents has been designed to ensure this is simply, quick and easy. Here all recipes are featured with their corresponding page number. Initially, it will take you a little to get used to, however once you become familiar with the layout you'll be able to "flick" straight to the page! Essentially, Part 2 and Part 3 act as reference points. Part 2 is where your recipes are featured, whilst Part 3 provides points of reference when performing the exercises set out in the Guide. At times you will find repetition – this is to ensure key points become second nature, whilst reaffirming form *and* technique parameters for functional movements to become commonplace throughout your 12 Week journey.

When it comes to time, the majority of *all* recipes take between 15-20 minutes to prepare. There are recipes that do take longer, however these are meat-based and thus a lengthened cooking time has been allowed. As for your *fitness* time commitment, your strength Guide has been designed to go for no more than 30 minutes, whilst your aerobic Guide has also ensured time is of the essence – primarily 30 minute based sessions feature.

The Guide is yours – it is *your tool* to hold in both hands and to take control *and* responsibility of your renewed lifestyle. At the start of every week it is recommended to read through your weekly commitments and to **highlight** your "what", "when" and "how" – refreshing Parts 2 and 3 as necessary.

Preparation is key – by going over your Guide consistently, this will afford you hindsight for the week ahead. This includes ensuring your *pantry is full* and that you have all the ingredients that you need to follow your nutrition, any given week. All recipes have been designed with the ingredients to appear first to allow your grocery lists to be that much easier. When it comes to fitness, all programs are *home-based* with the odd piece of equipment required. The majority of the time these "pieces" can be found around the home. However, by reading your weekly Guide prior to its implementation, this will allow you to ensure you have any necessary equipment to keep you on track.

It is highly recommended to highlight your Guide on a consistent basis. This simple method will allow your shopping lists to be instant, and your strength and aerobic commitments more refined with all commitments discussed *with you* opposed to do "this" then do "that" without knowing – the Guide wants you to know to ensure functional movement parameters prevail.

With all done and said – you're ready. If you've read Parts 1, 2 and 3, the 12 Week Journey is now at your fingertips to implement, apply and to most importantly, *enjoy* the journey, *enjoy* the process, you've now been given the *reins* towards a healthier *and* fitter you – because *you* deserve it!

But first...

This is where your 12 Week Journey becomes a reality and where you're going to put it into action. But before we "start" we need to put some *goals* in place – your *reason*. You already have this reason otherwise you wouldn't have made it this far. But I would like you to mould this reason with the "smartie" principle:

- Specific (more than a few words)
- Measurable (give your goal a time-frame, when do you want it?)
- Achievable (nothing is stopping you, it is in YOUR control to accomplish it)
- Realistic (something you can achieve i.e. if you want to circumnavigate the world, awesome! But, maybe not

tomorrow unless you've done all the training and planning necessary to take on such a feat)

- **T**ime (there is a time-frame, whether it be in 1 week, 1 month or 1 year, be "specific" in your timeline)
- **I**nteresting (something you want, something you want to "find out" whether you can, something you've always wanted to know and go after)
- **E**xciting (you think about it with the biggest smile, it gives you goosebumps knowing how you'll feel WHEN you achieve it)

Whether you have one goal or a dozen more, adhering to the "smartie" principle will set them alight. But first, write them down. Not on the computer, nor on your phone, but with pen and paper – write these goals down, write your *reason* down. It doesn't matter if these goals are to be achieved within the "12 Week" timeframe, or from a year from now, it is all about what you want to accomplish towards a healthier *and* fitter you.

Now that you have your *reason* (goals) in writing, it is your responsibility to read over them – *every night*. These goals act as your catalyst – to motivate you to keep going, to keep following the Guide, every step of the way. And you can. Over the next 12 Weeks there will be goals you will be able to *tick off* – be proud! There will be goals you don't quite reach, but *you will* – persist! And there will be weeks where you'll want to add to your goals, to your reason – please do! It is now your responsibility to keep your goals, your reason, in your back *or* front pocket, just like the tennis "ball" and enjoy the ride – here we go!

4.1 Week 1

FITNESS GUIDE:

	Mon	Tue	Wed	Thurs	Fri	Sat
AM	Strength		Strength		Strength	
PM	Aerobic	Aerobic		Aerobic	Aerobic	

STRENGTH:

1. Sit down on a chair or couch – but it's not to be touched. Take your time and make sure you are "popping" your backside out and that your knees do *not* go over your toes. Repeat 3 x 15 nice and slowly.
2. Lay down on the floor – on your back. Point your toes straight and your arms can stay by your side. Proceed to lift your feet off the ground while keeping your legs straight. Lift and hold for 3 seconds. Repeat 3 x 15 nice and slowly.
3. Find a table around hip height. Place hands spread a part on the ledge of the table. Move your feet backwards enough so when you lean into the table your chest will touch the same ledge your hands are on – keeping your back straight. Careful *not* to poke your backside into the air – you want to keep it tucked in. Proceed to lower yourself towards the ledge of the table but stop when your chest is in line with your elbows (so no, you don't want your chest touching the ledge). Repeat 3 x 15 nice and slowly.

Simple! Easy! That's all for this week.

AEROBIC:

1. You are going walking *with* a tennis ball! If you don't have a tennis ball, simply find a "ball" you can bounce.
2. Walk continuously for 30 minutes (15 minutes out, 15 minutes back) and consciously *bounce* the ball every 5 minutes for 1 minute. The last 5 minutes will not have a bounce at the end.

Done! Easy! Remember slow and steady is best to begin any form of exercise or program and to me mindful of your own unique build, health & fitness condition, and work within your fitness zone – you are competing with yourself, no one else.

NUTRITION GUIDE:

	SNACK	LUNCH	SNACK	DINNER	SNACK
m	Breakfast Freestyle	Fruit	Cabbage & Pickle Salad	Muffin	Carrot & Kale Salad	Cake!
t	Breakfast Freestyle	Dried Fruit	Masala Infused Chicken Stir-Fry	Smoothie	Lentil & Kale Salad	Muffin
w	Breakfast Freestyle	Nuts	Carrot &Beetroot Salad	Cake!	Tofu Salad	Smoothie
th	Breakfast Freestyle	Smoothie	Kale & Beetroot Salad	Nuts	Seasoned Fish	Fruit
f	Breakfast Freestyle	Muffin	Beetroot & Sprout Salad	Fruit	Bean & Sweet Potato Salad	Cake!

Weekend: active rest + food is fuel

4.2 Week 2

FITNESS GUIDE:

	Mon	Tue	Wed	Thurs	Fri	Sat
AM	Strength		Strength		Strength	
PM	Aerobic	Aerobic		Aerobic	Aerobic	

STRENGTH:

1. Find a wall and stand against it. Lower yourself just like you would be sitting on a chair – your back will be leaning against the wall and you're sitting on an "imaginary" chair. Stay in this position with your hands by your side (not to touch the wall) being careful that your knees are *not* over your toes. Hold for 1 minute. Repeat 3 times.

2. Lay down on the floor – on your back. Put your knees together in the air and "imagine" you are riding a bicycle. Keeping your back *flat* without any arch, pushing it against the floor. Repeat 3 x 15 cycles, slow and steady.

3. Find a skipping rope, or rope in general, sturdy enough to hold your own weight *and* long enough to "hook" around an item/object *heavier* than you. Now, be careful here! Place the object around a sturdy chair, for example, so you have both ends of the rope in either hand. Sit on the floor still holding onto the rope ends. Now you need to *pull* with the help of a few *wiggles* towards the item/object, gathering the loose rope ends in your hands as you go. Focus on the pulling part – keeping a *straight* back and with a slight bend at the knees – keeping your pulls between 15-20 (try not to sit too far away). Repeat pulling yourself towards the item/object (fridge, washing machine, car tire, or couch for example) 3 times.

Simple! Easy! That's all for this week.

AEROBIC:

1. You are going walking *with* the same tennis ball – again: use the ball from last week.
2. Walk continuously for 30 minutes (15 minutes out, 15 minutes back) and consciously *bounce* the ball every 5 minutes for 1 minute and then the following minute jog for 1 minute - at your own pace ensuring you can "last" the entire minute. Do your best. Go at your own pace – you want to last the *full* minute – but you want to make it count! The last 2 minutes are to finish with a 1 minute bounce then 1 minute jog, taking you to the 30 minutes.

Done! Easy! Remember slow and steady is best to begin any form of exercise or program and to be mindful of your own unique build, health & fitness condition, and work within your fitness zone - you are competing *with* yourself, no one else.

NUTRITION GUIDE:

		SNACK	LUNCH	SNACK	DINNER	SNACK
m	Breakfast Freestyle	Fruit	Cabbage & Broccoli Salad	Muffin	Potato & Kale Salad	Cake!
t	Breakfast Freestyle	Dried Fruit	Kale & Apple Salad	Smoothie	Vegetable Stir-Fry	Muffin
w	Breakfast Freestyle	Nuts	Lentil & Bean Mixed Salad	Cake!	Spiced Chicken Spinach Wrap	Smoothie
th	Breakfast Freestyle	Smoothie	Sauerkraut & Ricotta Salad	Nuts	Broccoli & Olive Pasta	Fruit
f	Breakfast Freestyle	Muffin	Pickle Pasta Salad	Fruit	Vitamin-Packed Spiced Soup	Cake!

Weekend: active rest + food is fuel

4.3 Week 3

FITNESS GUIDE:

	Mon	Tue	Wed	Thurs	Fri	Sat
AM	Strength		Strength		Strength	
PM	Aerobic	Aerobic		Aerobic	Aerobic	

STRENGTH:

1. Find a wall and stand against it. Lower yourself just like you would be sitting on a chair – your back will be leaning against the wall and you're sitting on an "imaginary" chair (again). Stay in this position with your hands by your side (careful with the wall) whilst being careful that your knees are *not* over your toes. Now *lift* one knee towards the sky – work within your range – count to 3 then place back on the floor. Do the opposite leg. Repeat 15 x per leg for 3 sets.
2. Lay down on the floor – on your back. Keeping your back *flat* without any arch, pushing it against the floor. Place your knees together and lift towards your belly-button (as close to as you can, within your limits). Place your feet back on the floor. Repeat 15 times x 3 sets.
3. Position yourself in the "push-up" position *but* with your knees on the floor. Keep your back straight and your backside *tucked* in. Go down for 1 count then when *raised* place one arm out in front (straight) for one-count – then place back down. Repeat the push-up action. On the way *up* place the opposite arm out in front (straight). Repeat 15 x for each arm x 3 sets.

Simple! Easy! That's all for this week.

AEROBIC:

1. You are walking with a tennis ball – again. You should have "your" ball of choice by now so I'm not going to remind you, it's your *reason* after all.

2. Walk continuously for 30 minutes (15 minutes out, 15 minutes back) whilst consciously holding onto the ball – every 3 minutes jog for 1 minute – at your *own pace* ensuring you can "last" the entire minute – keep the ball held in your hand. Do your best. Go at your own pace – you want to last the *full* minute, but you want to make it worth it! the last 2 minutes are to finish with a 2 minute jog – remembering you are competing with yourself, no one else. This will take you to your 30 minutes.

Done! Easy! Remember slow and steady is best to begin any form of exercise or program and to be mindful of your own unique build, health & fitness condition, and work within your fitness zone.

NUTRITION GUIDE:

		SNACK	LUNCH	SNACK	DINNER	SNACK
m	Breakfast Freestyle	Fruit	Zucchini & Avocado Salad	Muffin	Sweet Potato with Dried Fruit Salad	Cake!
t	Breakfast Freestyle	Dried Fruit	Kale & Sprout Salad	Smoothie	Spiced Chicken & Mushrooms	Muffin
w	Breakfast Freestyle	Nuts	Cabbage & Beetroot Salad	Cake!	Spinach & Salmon Salad	Smoothie
th	Breakfast Freestyle	Smoothie	Carrot & Kale Salad	Nuts	Mixed Spice Pumpkin Soup	Fruit
f	Breakfast Freestyle	Muffin	Cabbage & Olive Salad	Fruit	Sweet Potato Pasta Bake	Cake!

Weekend: active rest + food is fuel

4.4 Week 4

FITNESS GUIDE:

	Mon	Tue	Wed	Thurs	Fri	Sat
AM	Strength		Strength		Strength	
PM	Aerobic	Aerobic		Aerobic	Aerobic	

STRENGTH:

1. Stand upright with your feet shoulder width a part. Twist your body so your feet are pointing in one direction, aligned with one another with your hips centred. You are about to start doing *lunges*. Bend your front knee whilst a gentle bend remains in your back knee. Drop your back knee as close as you can to the floor *being careful* with your front knee – we don't want it to go beyond our toes. If it looks like you can't prevent this, widen your stance until it is comfortable. Now start – 2 lunges on one leg, then switch to the other leg and do 2 more. Repeat pattern 10 x 3.

2. Lay down on the floor – on your back. Point your toes forward and keep your arms by your side (palms upwards). Draw your feet towards your chest (bend at the knees to do this) and then hold for a 3 second count – slowly drop your legs back to the floor. Repeat 3 x 15.

3. You will need 2 x bottles that you can hold comfortably in your hands – you want the volume to be more than 1L. Once you have these *weights*, stand upright with one bottle in either hand. Keep your arms straight and push these out in front, slowly, on a 3 second count so that your arms are pointing towards the floor (creating a triangle between your arms and body). Now, draw the bottles back into your chest – this time bending at the arms so the bottles can touch your chest. Hold for 3 seconds and repeat – focusing on the "push" and "pull" motion. Repeat 3 x 15.

Simple! Easy! That's all for this week.

AEROBIC:

1. You are going walking with your ball, but this week we're going to pick up the pace. Going at your own speed, increase it by 20% – remembering this is your own pace and you're increasing *your* speed, no one else's.

2. Walk continuously for 30 minutes (15 minutes out, 15 minutes back) and consciously *hold onto* the ball – just like you are now accustomed. You are going to jog every second minute for 30 seconds. That means for every 1 minute 30 seconds you are walking, then the next 30 seconds you are jogging at an increase of 20% from your "normal" speed/pace. You can walk as slow as needed to recover from those 30 seconds you are pushing yourself to go that 20% faster – the objective is to increase your heart rate a little bit more this week. Again, working at your own pace and what is comfortable for you – no one else.

3. But what about the ball? Count to 5 and then bounce. Every 5 seconds bounce that ball. Narrow in on those 5 seconds and when the time comes to run, keep bouncing the ball every 5 seconds: that's 6 times when jogging, and 18 times when walking.

4. By going for 00.01.30 seconds walking, and then 00.00.30 seconds jogging, this will take you to your 30 minutes.

Done! Easy! Remember slow and steady is best to begin any form of exercise or program and to be mindful of your own unique build, health and fitness condition, and work within your fitness zone.

NUTRITION GUIDE:

	Breakfast	SNACK	LUNCH	SNACK	DINNER	SNACK
m	Breakfast Freestyle	Fruit	Moroccan Inspired Cabbage Salad	Muffin	Sweet Potato & Cabbage Salad	Cake!
t	Breakfast Freestyle	Dried Fruit	Green Bean Salad	Smoothie	Jaw Dropping Tofu Burgers	Nuts
w	Breakfast Freestyle	Muffin	Spring Salad	Cake!	Cabbage & Mushroom Salad	Smoothie
th	Breakfast Freestyle	Smoothie	Cabbage & Beans	Nuts	Indian Infused Siru Curry	Fruit
f	Breakfast Freestyle	Muffin	Carrot & Broccoli Salad	Fruit	Potato & Avocado Salad	Cake!

Weekend: active rest + food is fuel

4.5 Week 5

FITNESS GUIDE:

	Mon	Tue	Wed	Thurs	Fri	Sat
AM	Strength	Strength		Strength	Strength	
PM	Aerobic	Aerobic		Aerobic	Aerobic	Aerobic

STRENGTH:

1. This week we're going to do a circuit – but it is *your* circuit, at *your* pace, at *your* own level. We're mixing things up to make it quick and simple whilst maintaining your progress and results. First we're going to lunge – be careful that your front knee doesn't go over your toes and that your back knee stays off the floor – ever so slightly.

2. Maintain a solid posture with your shoulders back and belly-button tucked in nice and tight. Second we're going to plank – elbows on the ground in an upside down "V" shape, your toes should be supporting your weight whilst your backside feels like it is sticking up in the air! Now, lower your backside so your back is *firm* and straight. Remove any arches from your back whilst being careful not to "sink in" nor "poke" upwards. Third we're going to drop down to our knees from the plank position, keeping a straight back, whilst rising onto our hands so we create a 90-degree angle between out elbows and the floor...yes, you're doing to do *push-ups*.

3. For the more advanced, you can stay on your toes – remembering to work at your level. Okay, now you have the Three exercises for this week's circuit. Yes, just three – quick and simple!

Here's what we're going to do:

1. Lunge left leg x 15
2. Plank 30 seconds
3. Push-up x 5
4. Lunge right leg x 15
5. Plank 45 seconds
6. Push-up x 10
7. Lunge alternating legs x 20
8. Plank 60 seconds
9. Push-up x 15
10. Lunge left leg x 15
11. Plank 45 seconds
12. Push-up x 10
13. Lunge right leg x 15
14. Plank 30 seconds
15. Push-up x 5

Simple! Easy! That's all for this week.

AEROBIC:

1. This week we're going to focus on distance.
2. The goal? Let's see how far you can travel in the space of 30 minutes alternating between walking *and* jogging. This means *stop* and *start* for 30 minutes. Yes, you're going to use the ball again and *every* time you start/stop jogging and/or walking, you're going to bounce the ball for the number of minutes you have jogged or for the number of minutes you have walked. for example, if you're able to jog for 3 minutes, bounce the ball for 3 minutes. If you walk for 10 minutes before you start to job, bounce the ball for 10 minutes *before* you start to jog.
3. The goal? Keep going! Keep walking...keep jogging for the full 30 minutes and *track* your distance. You want to see how far you have come! How far can you go in 30 minutes? Good luck!

Done! Easy! Remember slow and steady is best to begin any form of exercise or program and to be mindful of your own unique build, health and fitness condition, and work within your fitness zone.

NUTRITION GUIDE:

		SNACK	LUNCH	SNACK	DINNER	SNACK
m	Breakfast Freestyle	Fruit	Celery & Beetroot Salad	Muffin	Lightly Spiced Roast Chicken	Cake!
t	Breakfast Freestyle	Dried Fruit	Bean & Sweet Potato Salad	Smoothie	Cabbage & Mushroom Pasta Salad	Muffin
w	Breakfast Freestyle	Nuts	Chicken & Coriander Salad	Cake!	Coconut Pickled Salad	Smoothie
th	Breakfast Freestyle	Smoothie	Sweet Potato, Spinach & Rice Salad	Nuts	Tofu Chilli Salad	Fruit
f	Breakfast Freestyle	Muffin	Cabbage & Pickle Salad	Fruit	Jaw Dropping Chicken Burgers	Cake!

Weekend: active rest + food is fuel

4.6 Week 6

FITNESS GUIDE:

	Mon	Tue	Wed	Thurs	Fri	Sat
AM	Strength	Strength		Strength	Strength	
PM	Aerobic	Aerobic		Aerobic	Aerobic	Aerobic

STRENGTH:

1. Progressing from last week, you're going to continue with the circuit designed for you – unique to your *level* and your own *pace*.
2. Remembering to keep a solid posture: tight core and shoulders "back and down" so you feel locked-in or rather tucked-in and *strong*.
3. Now you're going to *squat* ensuring your knees do *not* pass your toes. At the bottom of the squat, hold for 5 seconds and then lift.
4. Keeping the locked-in posture, lean at a 90-degree angle against a bench – "push-up" position whilst *leaning*. From here, set yourself up like you would be doing a push-up, maintaining you tucked position. Now proceed to "push" through your *left* arm, then *both* arms, then your *right* arm.
5. Next, holding onto that posture, you're going to need a milk carton *or* object you can carry comfortably with both hands, but heavy enough not to want to hold onto it for more than a minute. From here you're going to grasp the object with both hands, standing *tall*. Now, rotate to your left. We want to do a full semi-circle – what we do *not* want is to twist past the side of our body. Once rotated to your left, rotate to the right and then back to centre nice and slow. Take 3 seconds to go from left, 3 seconds to centre, 3 seconds to go to right, then 3 seconds to go back to centre.

Here we go:

1. Squat x 15
2. Push x 15
3. Rotate x 15
4. Push x 20
5. Rotate x 20
6. Squat x 20
7. Rotate x 10
8. Squat x 10
9. Push x 10

Simple! Easy! That's all for this week.

AEROBIC:

1. Last week we worked on distance so this week we are going to work on going that little bit quicker...that little bit faster...that little bit longer! Keep using *your* (tennis) ball.

2. You are going to be conscious of bouncing this ball *before* you sprint and *after* you sprint.

3. Here's how you're going to break-down this week's 30 minutes:
   - Walk 2 minutes.
   - Jog 1 minute.
   - Sprint 30 seconds.

4. Now, when you're sprinting be mindful to go at your pace. When jogging, you want to just go lightly so you're not "over doing" it, allowing yourself to sprint for the following 30 seconds.

5. Overall you're going to get in 8 sprints, whilst the remaining 2 minutes will be for jogging to cool-down your body.

6. At the end of the 30 minutes be mindful of how far you were able to travel and cover in these 30 minutes and towards the end of the week, look back on how far you've come!

Done! Easy! Remember slow and steady is best to begin any form of exercise or program and to be mindful of your own unique build, health and fitness condition, and work within your fitness zone.

NUTRITION GUIDE:

		SNACK	LUNCH	SNACK	DINNER	SNACK
m	Breakfast Freestyle	Fruit	Celery & Beetroot Salad	Muffin	Lightly Spiced Roast Chicken	Cake!
t	Breakfast Freestyle	Dried Fruit	Bean & Sweet Potato Salad	Smoothie	Cabbage & Mushroom Pasta Salad	Muffin
w	Breakfast Freestyle	Nuts	Chicken & Coriander Salad	Cake!	Coconut Pickled Salad	Smoothie
th	Breakfast Freestyle	Smoothie	Sweet Potato, Spinach & Rice Salad	Nuts	Tofu Chilli Salad	Fruit
f	Breakfast Freestyle	Muffin	Cabbage & Pickle Salad	Fruit	Jaw Dropping Chicken Burgers	Cake!

Weekend: active rest + food is fuel

4.7 Week 7

FITNESS GUIDE:

	Mon	Tue	Wed	Thurs	Fri	Sat
AM	Strength	Strength		Strength	Strength	
PM	Aerobic	Aerobic		Aerobic	Aerobic	Aerobic

STRENGTH + AEROBIC

This week we're going to mix things up. Besides your "ball" you've been holding onto the past few weeks, this week you're also going to need a skipping rope. It doesn't matter what type of rope you have, just as long as you can skip with it!

So what are we doing? We are mixing it up and putting your *strength + aerobic* all in one this week. That means you can do half the program in the morning and the other at night if you're short on time, or you can "kill two birds with one stone" as the saying goes!

Here we go:

1. Use your skipping rope to do 50 skips. Whilst skipping, stand *tall* and do your best not to lean forward.
2. Next, you're going to squat down so the back of your thighs are touching your calves – in a "frog" position. Once down you will hold the count for 3 seconds – bouncing the ball for those 3 seconds – then *jump* up as high as you can. Repeat the frog jump x 15.
3. Pick up the skipping rope again and do 3 x 25 skips. After each set of 25 skips bounce the ball the number of times you were able to skip straight – without error.
4. Find a wall to stand against. Lean into the wall so your hands are touching the wall yet your body is on a slight angle. Imagine that you are *pushing* the wall slowly, but surely. This is your starting position. From here you are going to lean right into the wall so your head is a few centimetres away from it in which then you are going

to use your *power* to *push* off the wall. Keep your balance intact and step back with your leading leg to counteract the force. Repeat x 15.

5. Use your skipping rope this time to skip 3 x 50 and in between sets you will do 10 x frog jumps and 10 x wall pushes.
6. This time pick up the pace on your skipping and do 5 x 25 skips. Between each set you will do 20 x frog jumps followed by 20 x wall pushes.
7. To finish, you're going to hold onto the ball and bounce it every 10 steps – jogging. You are going to run for 100 bounces then walk for 1 minute. Continue the 100 bounces followed by the 1 minute walk for 10 minutes.

Done! This week's program is touch, but it is also made *super* easy by combining both your *strength* + *aerobic* to show that irrespective of time, there is always time for your health – thus fitness.

Remember slow and steady is best to begin any form of exercise or program and to be mindful of your own unique build, health & fitness condition, and work within your fitness zone.

Simple! Easy! That's all for this week.

NUTRITION GUIDE:

		SNACK	LUNCH	SNACK	DINNER	SNACK
m	Breakfast Freestyle	Fruit	Lentil & Kale Salad	Muffin	Seasoned Fish	Cake!
t	Breakfast Freestyle	Dried Fruit	Zucchini & Avocado Salad	Smoothie	Pickle Pasta Salad	Muffin
w	Breakfast Freestyle	Nuts	Carrot & Kale Salad	Cake!	Sweet Potato Pasta Bake	Smoothie
th	Breakfast Freestyle	Smoothie	Cabbage & Olive Salad	Nuts	Carrot & Beetroot Salad	Fruit
f	Breakfast Freestyle	Muffin	Kale & Beetroot Salad	Fruit	Masala Infused Chicken Stir-Fry	Cake!

Weekend: active rest + food is fuel

4.8 Week 8

FITNESS GUIDE:

	Mon	Tue	Wed	Thurs	Fri	Sat
AM	Strength	Strength		Strength	Strength	
PM	Aerobic	Aerobic		Aerobic	Aerobic	Aerobic

STRENGTH:

Seven weeks have now past which means if you're reading this, you're up to week *eight* and your fitness base has improved near ten-fold in this short time! This week you've some important questions to ask yourself:

1. How far have I come?
2. How much farther do I want to go?
3. What pushes me, why am I doing this, and how do I feel? These link right into your goals and we have reached a point now where your *goals,* your *reason,* become paramount – they're going to either keep you going, or you'll *stop*. I want the *best* for *you* – which means this week your "homework" is to write down every training day 3 *goals* – these can be reaffirmed from your "set" *goals* and *reason* in place, or entirely new! Keep going until you have a total of 10 *specific* goals that follow the "smartie" principle (see Outline).

So now you're wondering, what's in store to push you that little but further this week? We're going to build our endurance – anaerobically: we're going to see "how many" we can do each day and set our individual benchmarks – at your *level* and your own *pace*. This week you're going to need to remember all of our "cues" for each exercise. If you've come this far, chronologically, you will be fine! If, however you have jumped a few weeks, revise Part 3 to ensure you're aware of **technique 101** parameters to near-eliminate the risk of injury.

Until you reach your max (i.e. can no longer do any more):

1. Lunges – how many can you do before your posture gives way? [*keeping our shoulders tucked back and an upright stance, ensuring your front knee does not go over your toes*]

2. Squats – how many can you do before your legs won't bend? [*keeping your shoulders tucked back and an upright stance, ensuring your front knee does not go over your toes and that your posture allows you to "stick" your backside out whilst keeping it down*]

3. Curls with "milk bottles" – how many can you do with both arms? [*ensuring an upright stance is kept and you don't start "swinging" your arms", whilst keeping your elbows nice and close to your sides*]

4. Pulls, on floor with rope – how far can you pull yourself? [*keeping your shoulders back and down, leaning forward through the hips, how many pulls can you do of your own body weight? reposition yourself every time you do a full round of "pulls" until you can do no more*]

5. Angled push-ups – how many can you do before your elbows won't allow you to go any further? [*leaning against a bench/table, ensuring you have good posture and that your belly-button is drawn towards your spine*]

Simple! Easy! That's all for this week.

AEROBIC:

It has been seven weeks and come week eight it is time to see *how far we can run*...period!

1. This week's challenge thus is to see how *far* you can run and how *long* you can run for. We're still going to stick to the 30 minute rule – if you can run for 30 minutes straight you're going to need to pick up *your* own pace and *your* own speed to challenge yourself at a quicker pace/speed to see if "that" pace can be kept for the same amount of time.

2. As for the tennis ball – we still want it...but this week your *ball* plays an important role – a powerful role: every time you think of slowing, every time you doubt you can go that little bit further, remember *everything* you have done, everything you have been through to get to this point, and how "that" ball has been with you every step of the way – knowing that you're capable of going that one step further.

3. The challenge? You're going to push yourself a little bit further than you ever have over these past seven weeks and you're going to find out how far you've come, and how far you're capable of going!

Done! Easy! *I'd love to know how you've been progressing over these past now eight weeks – please let me know over on Instagram or Twitter so I can celebrate your progress with you!*

NUTRITION GUIDE:

		SNACK	LUNCH	SNACK	DINNER	SNACK
m	Breakfast Freestyle	Fruit	Kale & Sprout Salad	Muffin	Sweet Potato with Dried Fruit Salad	Cake!
t	Breakfast Freestyle	Dried Fruit	Potato & Kale Salad	Smoothie	Broccoli & Olive Pasta	Muffin
w	Breakfast Freestyle	Nuts	Carrot & Kale Salad	Cake!	Spinach & Salmon Salad	Smoothie
th	Breakfast Freestyle	Smoothie	Cabbage & Broccoli Salad	Nuts	Mixed Spice Pumpkin Soup	Fruit
f	Breakfast Freestyle	Muffin	Green Bean Salad	Fruit	Indian Infused Siru Curry	Cake!

Weekend: active rest + food is fuel

4.9 Week 9

FITNESS GUIDE:

	Mon	Tue	Wed	Thurs	Fri	Sat
AM	Strength	Strength		Strength	Strength	Strength
PM	Aerobic	Aerobic		Aerobic	Aerobic	Aerobic

STRENGTH:

We've now come to week nine and we're going to mix things up again. A big focus this week is going to be on flexibility and controlled movements. To begin with, you're going to need a skipping rope briefly to get yourself warmed up.

Skip 25 x 4 sets and then you can start!

Here we go:

1. Stand upright against a wall until your forearm is leaning against the wall (vertically) whilst your body is aside. Now, push your chest forwards slightly until you feel that stretch (in the chest vicinity – stretching your "pec" muscle). Hold for 30 seconds each side.
2. Drop down to the floor and do 8 x push-ups with a focus on *control* – use your knees if you need whilst keeping your belly-button is kept drawn towards your spine.
3. Repeat chest stretch and hold for 30 seconds.
4. Drop down and do 12 x push-ups.
5. Repeat chest stretch and hold for 30 seconds.
6. Drop down and do 15 x push-ups

Done! That is, your chest...

1. Stand tall with your feet extended "more than" shoulder width apart – then proceed to bend at the hips, leaning down trying to get your hands to touch the ground – widen your stance if necessary. Hold for 30 seconds (being careful to raise slowly to ensure the

blood doesn't rush straight back to your head!). Then, lean to your *left* and hold for 30 seconds. Then, lean to your *right* and hold for 30 seconds.

2. Stand tall then proceed to bend your knees, readying to lunge. Now, do 10 x consecutive controlled lunges followed by 10 x *jump lunges*: these are new – the difference is that when you go "down" you're going to "jump" into the next lunge, rather than slowly transition.

3. Repeat *all* groin stretches

4. Lunge x 15 followed by Jump Lunges x 15

5. Repeat *all* groin stretches

6. Lunges x 20 followed by Jump Lunges x 20

Your legs are now done!

1. Slowly drop down to the floor and lay on your back. Keeping your back on the floor, twist your right leg over your body so it is stretched over to the left side of your body (bending at the knee). Hold for 30 seconds then repeat with your left leg.

2. Keep your toes pointed straight and your back on the floor, slowly raise your feet *off* the ground. Keeping your legs straight and your arms by your side, lift your feet/toes as far off the ground as you're comfortable (aiming for a range of 10cm's to 30cm's) – hold for 30 seconds and then lower your feet to the ground.

3. Repeat leg stretch trying to push the stretch a little deeper. Hold for 45 seconds either side.

4. Laying on your back, again, point your toes and let them sit between 10-30cm's off the ground and then proceed to "scissor kick" (up/down toes without touching the floor) for 45 seconds.

5. Repeat leg stretch – going deeper into the muscle. Hold for 1 minute.

6. Repeat scissor kick whilst keeping your back flat on the floor – continue for 1 minute and then lower feet slowly to the ground.

Your core is done!

Repeat *all* stretches from the top, holding for 30 seconds each and then you are finished! Simple! Easy! That's all for this week.

AEROBIC:

1. For week nine we are going to keep it as simple as it comes – this week you're going to run for 8 minutes then walk for 2 minutes. Simple! But your challenge is to find your "pace" that will allow you to *keep going* for those 8 minutes.

2. Once you have run for 8 minutes you are then going to walk for 2 minutes. During these minutes you're going to need your ball. Slow your *heart rate* down by bouncing the ball for *every* heartbeat. If you were able to go "slow and steady" and not wear yourself out, you will be able to keep the ball bouncing in line with your heart rate (beat) – but, if the beat is too fast, slow yourself until the ball can fall in sync with your heart beat (rate).

3. You have 3 sets of running – the 1st is slow and steady, the 2nd is a little quicker, being mindful of your heart rate (the challenge is to ensure you won't stop, but to also know you have a *full* 2 minutes to *recover*), whilst 3rd is that little bit quicker, controlling your run (we don't want to be flapping and swinging our arms all over the place) – then walk it out through to the end, capping off those 30 minutes.

4. Be mindful of the ball's bounce and if your *heart rate* at the beginning of your runs has been maintained, or if it is higher. Either way it doesn't matter, but if it is the same – this is telling you that you didn't push yourself hard enough – you were (and are) capable of more than you think!

Done! Easy! *I'd love to know how you've been progressing over these past now nine weeks – please let me know over on Twitter or Instagram so I can celebrate your progress with you!*

NUTRITION GUIDE:

		SNACK	LUNCH	SNACK	DINNER	SNACK
m	Breakfast Freestyle	Fruit	Moroccan Inspired Cabbage Salad	Muffin	Spiced Chicken & Mushrooms	Cake!
t	Breakfast Freestyle	Dried Fruit	Cabbage & Beetroot Salad	Smoothie	Vegetable Stir-Fry	Muffin
w	Breakfast Freestyle	Nuts	Celery & Beetroot Salad	Cake!	Potato & Avocado Salad	Smoothie
th	Breakfast Freestyle	Smoothie	Sweet Potato & Cabbage Salad	Nuts	Chicken & Coriander Salad	Fruit
f	Breakfast Freestyle	Muffin	Spring Salad	Fruit	Jaw Dropping Tofu Burgers	Cake!

Weekend: active rest + food is fuel

4.10 Week 10

FITNESS GUIDE:

	Mon	Tue	Wed	Thurs	Fri	Sat
AM	Strength	Strength		Strength	Strength	Strength
PM	Aerobic	Aerobic		Aerobic	Aerobic	Aerobic

STRENGTH:

Time has flown by and when you're consciously working towards a goal, in this case a *lifestyle* underpinned by *reason*, time is to be treasured. Over the past nine weeks, this "time" may not have previously been put to work – you have begun to realize, and it has been reaffirmed, that by working towards a healthier *and* fitter version of you, not only physically have you seen changes, but also emotional and behavioural too. This is an incredible stage to be at and to realize why time spent on *you* is time well spent - the ripple effect becomes apparent with your *optimal wellbeing* shifting for the better without even consciously being aware of what or how it is evolving – it just is by means of putting your plan, this Guide, into action.

Take a few minutes to digest the changes that have presented themselves over the course of the past nine weeks. Go over your goals initially set and those that have been "ticked" and those you're continuously working towards. And remember, your *reason* for implementing this Guide.

Add to it. What is something you are yet to achieve that you would thrive off achieving? Align it with the "smartie" principle and lay it out for you to work towards achieving, with this week as your catalyst.

This week you are going to rely on your *prior* knowledge and understanding of what you have been doing to ensure you have been applying the **technique 101** parameters. This week has been stripped back and simplified – you are going to rely on yourself, mostly, to execute this week's program: as you *interpret* it.

1. Skipping rope – 5 x 25 skips
2. Legs: couch squats – 3 x 20
3. Lunge – 3 x 12 with every 4th lunge to be *jumped*
4. Squat *hold* – 3 x 45 seconds
   > Each set is to be done once and then move onto the next exercise – this way you will repeat Couch Squats, Lunges then Squats *three* times.
5. Back: tie your *rope* to a heavy object – heavy enough so it will not move when you pull the rope. You will need the rope length to be at least 3 meters long.
6. Sitting on the floor, tiled area preferred to you don't get "carpet burn" you are going to *hold* the rope with both hands (think: tug-of-war) and you are going to *pull* yourself towards the opposite end of the rope. Be mindful that this length is to be *no more* than 4 meters (ideally 3 meters in length).
7. Now you need a heavy object that you can roll or push. Making sure you have between 10-20 metres to roll or push the object. If you do not have that kind of space, don't worry. All you then need to do is to compensate by going back-and-forth rather than one-way.
8. You are now going to roll or push your object for 3 x 15 "heavy" pushes (or rolls). Alternatively, depending on your object you can roll or push for 45 seconds. You *choose*.
9. Repeat rope pull and roll/push exercises alternatively until 3 sets of each is complete.
10. Chest: table pushes – 3 x 15
11. Standing against a wall with your arms in the push "down" (up) position – push *back* (against) with *power*! Repeat 3 x 15
12. Push-up position: attempt to JUMP with your hands every second *push* (up). Repeat 3 x 15
13. To end: sitting on the floor with your knees bent, grab 2 x *milk bottles* or similar. Hold these in your hands.

Keeping a tight core, *twist* slowly to your left, then slowly to your *right*, then back to the *centre,* slowly. Emphasis here is on a "controlled" movement. Repeat 2 x 25 sets.

Simple! Easy! That's all for this week.

AEROBIC:

Let's mix things up! The time has come to show you how fitness *is* fun whilst ensuring our movements are with intention all the whilst being controlled.

This week you're going to need a *skateboard*! There is a very good chance that you do *not* have one, but if you are a typical "young adult", there is a good chance you know someone who *does* own one. And not to worry, all you need is a basic board, nothing fancy!

1. With your skateboard, keeping it stationary, you are going to do "toe taps" – whereby you lift your toes up interchangeably, slightly touching the board, then switching between feet – as quick as you can! Controlled "taps" are emphasised as to not move the board. 6 x 30 seconds with a 10 second break for each set (taking you to 4 minutes).
2. With *one* leg, *skate* slowly, lifting your foot that isn't on the board nice and *slow*. Do this for 2 minutes and then *change* to the opposite leg for 2 minutes (we are now up to 8 minutes).
3. Grab the ball and with one leg slowly kick (skate) until you have kicked x 10 – with each kick you will *bounce* the ball once. Change legs and kick x 10 allowing 1 minute for each leg (we are now up to 10 minutes).
4. Working on your balance *and* control, nice and slowly on your leg of choice (where you feel at your steadiest), free-skate for the next 2 minutes (taking you to 12 minutes).
5. Hop off your board and do *toe taps* – 6 x 30 seconds with a 10 seconds break in between (we are now up to 16 minutes).
6. For the remaining 14 minutes you have a *choice*: you can skate for *half* the remaining time (7 minutes longer) *or* you can begin your *long run*. Yes, for the remaining time you are going to *run* at your *own* pace ensuring

you can last for the *entire* time without walking. For every 30 steps counted with one leg (foot strike) bounce the *ball* once.

7. Whether you choose to run for 7 minutes or 14 minutes, one is working more so on your balance, the other with an emphasis on your aerobic capacity. If you do choose the 7 minutes, you will simply push yourself a little bit extra to allow your heart rate to catch up!

Done! Easy! *I'd love to know how you've been progressing over these past ten weeks - please let me know over on Instagram or Twitter so I can celebrate your progress with you!*

NUTRITION GUIDE:

	SNACK	LUNCH	SNACK	DINNER	SNACK
m	Breakfast Freestyle	Fruit	Coconut Pickled Salad	Muffin	Tofu Chilli Salad	Cake!
t	Breakfast Freestyle	Dried Fruit	Sweet Potato with Dried Fruit Salad	Smoothie	Cabbage & Beans	Muffin
w	Breakfast Freestyle	Nuts	Carrot & Broccoli Salad	Cake!	Jaw Dropping Chicken Burgers	Smoothie
th	Breakfast Freestyle	Smoothie	Cabbage & Pickle Salad	Nuts	Sweet Potato, Spinach & Rice Salad	Fruit
f	Breakfast Freestyle	Muffin	Cabbage & Mushroom Pasta Salad	Fruit	Masala Infused Chicken Stir-Fry	Cake!

Weekend: active rest + food is fuel

4.11 Week 11

FITNESS GUIDE:

	Mon	Tue	Wed	Thurs	Fri	Sat
AM	Strength	Strength		Strength	Strength	Strength
PM	Aerobic	Aerobic		Aerobic	Aerobic	Aerobic

STRENGTH:

It is time to work that little bit harder, to push yourself that little bit further, and to tread that little bit faster. This week's program is *fast*, it'll be *challenging*, but if you've done the work up until now, you'll *breeze* through it with your *endorphins* getting you over the line.

Again, using your prior knowledge whilst using Part 3 as a point of reference, here we go:

1. Walking lunges with milk bottles x 15 each leg (30 total)
2. Walking lunges with milk bottles – backwards x 15 each leg (30 total)
3. Burpees x 15 – 1 set – repeat all 3 exercises 3 times
4. Hang rope over sturdy object that will hold your own body weight. Please take caution to ensure the object can hold your own weight. You are going to hook the rope over the object so you can pull yourself *up* towards the object whilst hovering off the ground i.e. a 45-degree angle. Pull yourself up x 15
5. Roll over and complete 15 x push-ups
6. Roll back over and pull yourself up and *hold* for a 15 second count
7. Roll over and complete 15 x push-ups
8. Roll back over and pull yourself up and on your way back down *count* to 15 seconds *slowly* lowering yourself back down
9. Roll back over and complete 15 x push-ups
10. Lay on the ground and set yourself into the *plank* position (push-up position but with your body supported by your elbows with your forearms horizontal on the ground).

Ensure your belly-button is tucked in tightly and that your back is nice and *straight* with minimal arch in your back (note: your abdominal muscles are to work here, *not* your back – so if your back begins to weaken you will need to straighten your back, being careful not to curve – think *straight* as a plank). Hold plank position for 30 seconds

11. Roll over and complete 30 leg cycles (air cycling)
12. Roll back over and hold plank position for 45 seconds
13. Roll over and lay on the ground – lift your legs off the ground between 20-30cm's and hold for 60 seconds
14. Roll back over and hold plank position for 60 seconds
15. Roll over and scissor kick for 60 seconds
16. Then: 5 x jump lunges
17. 5 x push-ups
18. 5 x burpees
19. 5 x rope pulls
20. Repeat x 3 and you're done!

Simple! Easy! That's all for this week.

AEROBIC:

The time has come for us to go harder, further and faster. This week we are going to *sprint* and *jog*. You will need your skateboard again and as always, your *ball*.

Set out a 100m running track/path/area/section. This week you will be running up and down this area. Ideally, it will be *smooth* as you will need to be able to sprint, jog, and *skate* up and down this 100m track/path/area/section.

Holding onto your ball:

1. Jog for 100m x 3
2. Skate 100m x 1
3. Sprint 50m then jog the remaining 50m
4. Sprint 75m then jog the remaining 25m
5. Skate 100m x 1

(allowing 5 minutes total to this point)

6. Water break (1 minute)
7. Jog for 100m x 1
8. Sprint for 100m x 1
9. Jog for 50m then sprint for 50m
10. Skate for 100m
11. Sprint for 100m
12. Jog for 150m then sprint for 50m
13. Jog for 50m then sprint for 150m
14. Skate for 100m

(allowing 14 minutes total to this point)

15. Water break (1 minute)
16. Jog for 300m
17. Skate for 100m
18. Sprint for 25m, then jog for 25m, then sprint for 25m, then jog for 25m

19. Sprint for 50m then jog for 150m
20. Sprint for 100m
21. Skate for 100m

(allowing 23 minutes total to this point)

22. Water break (1 minute)
23. Keeping an eye on the time now, you are going to jog for 1 minute, then sprint for 15 seconds, jog for 15 seconds, then sprint for 30 seconds.
24. Jog for 30 seconds, sprint for 30 seconds, jog for 30 seconds, and then sprint for 30 seconds followed by a final skate for 2 minutes.

Done! Easy! Make sure you drink enough water once you're done after having worked harder, gone further, and ran faster! *I'd love to know how you've been progressing over these past eleven weeks and how your journey as a whole has evolved - please let me know over on Instagram or Twitter so I can celebrate your progress with you!*

NUTRITION GUIDE:

	Breakfast	SNACK	LUNCH	SNACK	DINNER	SNACK
m	Breakfast Freestyle	Fruit	Green Bean Salad	Muffin	Mixed Spice Pumpkin Soup	Cake!
t	Breakfast Freestyle	Dried Fruit	Sauerkraut & Ricotta Salad	Smoothie	Broccoli & Olive Pasta	Muffin
w	Breakfast Freestyle	Nuts	Cabbage & Olive Salad	Cake!	Lightly Spiced Roast Chicken	Smoothie
th	Breakfast Freestyle	Smoothie	Potato & Avocado Salad	Nuts	Sweet Potato, Spinach & Rice Salad	Fruit
f	Breakfast Freestyle	Muffin	Tofu Salad	Fruit	Indian Infused Siru Curry	Cake!

Weekend: active rest + food is fuel

4.12 Week 12

FITNESS GUIDE:

	Mon	Tue	Wed	Thurs	Fri	Sat
AM	Strength	Strength		Strength	Strength	Strength
PM	Aerobic	Aerobic		Aerobic	Aerobic	Aerobic

STRENGTH + AEROBIC:

It is upon us: the final week of your renewed and revamped *lifestyle* Guide. This week you're going put in everything left in the tank – show yourself what you're truly made of, whilst putting to work the healthier, fitter and *stronger* you!

To finish your 12 Week Guide we have grouped together for the final time your strength *and* aerobic programs in one. But before you get underway, it's time to reflect on how far you have come – re-address the "smartie" principle and this week you're going to endeavour to *tick-off* as many of those remaining *goals* as possible! Yes, you *can* do it, you *are* capable, and if you've come this far (which you *have*), you have already put in the hard yards. So, let's finish *strong*!

What you'll need:

1. Skipping rope.
2. Tube Rope (plyo-band – available at your nearest sporting store or physiotherapist; if you are unable to get your hands on one, use an old pair of "stretch" pants (jeans will provide the best resistance) otherwise *lean* your body into the movements using your skipping rope, "moving" your body with each movement in contrast to placing resistance on the bands (like you will, herein).
3. Tire (or *safe* heavy object you are able to move, flip, push, pull – safely).

Here we go:

1. Speed-skipping 10 x 10 (i.e. as fast as you can go!)
2. Lay tire (or object) on the ground and *flip* back-and-forth 3 x 12
3. Place tube rope around pole at chest height with your back to the pole (ends straight, *not* flimsy). Grab each end of the tube rope in separate hands then *press* forward like a standing *push-up* 3 x 12
4. Casual Skipping x 100

(allowing 10 minutes total including rest stops)

5. Go back to tire and *flip* back-and-forth (placing your hands underneath to push upwards) 3 x 12
6. Go back to the pole and grab each end of the tube rope using both hands - this time whilst *facing* the pole. Pull the tube rope towards you (until your elbows are in line with your body) 3 x 12
7. Speed-skipping 25 x 3
8. Jump lunges x 10
9. Burpees x 10
10. Squat hold for 30 seconds
11. Repeat *all* (7 to 10) x 3
12. Go back to pole and stand sideways (*activate* your core by drawing your belly-button towards your spine, maintaining this stance throughout). Using one hand, grab the tube rope with *one* hand and pull towards your *centre* (starting with your arm slightly bent with some *tension* already on the tube rope) – do 12 reps then change hands and repeat until you have done 3 x 12

(allowing 25 minutes total including rests)

13. Now it's time to grab your ball and *jog*: 15 minutes straight (aim to go at your fastest, yet steadiest pace, bouncing the ball every *90* steps you take)

(40 minutes complete)

14. Speed-skipping 25 x 3
15. Sprint runs: 50m sprint – 50m jog – 50m walk – 100m sprint – 150m jog – 50m walk – 200m jog – 100m sprint – 50m jog – 50m walk – 150m sprint
16. Fast jog – 5 minutes (bouncing the ball every *90* steps)
17. Casual skipping 3 x 50

(allowing 20 minutes including rest)

Done! You made it and I am so incredibly proud of you. This week presented the toughest of *all* weeks and relied on your *newly* acquired strength, physicality *and* mental toughness. Albeit 12 Weeks ago this was unfathomed. You did it and here on in, you *are* capable of continuously pushing towards the *next* healthier, fitter and stronger version of you – controlling and securing your *optimal wellbeing* for the years to come.

NUTRITION GUIDE:

		SNACK	LUNCH	SNACK	DINNER	SNACK
m	Breakfast Freestyle	Fruit	Kale & Apple Salad	Muffin	Spinach & Salmon Salad	Cake!
t	Breakfast Freestyle	Dried Fruit	Kale & Sprout Salad	Smoothie	Seasoned Chicken	Muffin
w	Breakfast Freestyle	Nuts	Zucchini & Avocado Salad	Cake!	Cabbage & Mushroom Pasta Salad	Smoothie
th	Breakfast Freestyle	Smoothie	Cabbage & Broccoli Salad	Nuts	Lentil & Bean Mixed Salad	Fruit
f	Breakfast Freestyle	Muffin	Sweet Potato with Dried Fruit Salad	Fruit	Sweet Potato Pasta Bake	Cake!

Weekend: active rest + food is fuel

Closing thoughts

Simplified, refined and easy to execute. This 12 Week Journey isn't, nor ever will be about overcomplicating or increased time consumption – it's a *lifestyle* improvement. Lifestyle changes are adaptable, time-efficient, *and* give you the reins to control and take responsibility for the restored and rejuvenated *you* – the commitment embedded within Part 4.

Functional movement fitness is something you have for life. You've learned the ropes, you've been guided through "how" to perform these movements, allowing you to take them wherever your renewed lifestyle choose.

Freestyle nutrition is on your terms. You've learned "how" to create in a simplified and refined way – cooking or meal preparation isn't complicated, its tangible! You have the tools to take you, too, wherever your renewed lifestyle chooses – no holding back.

Then there was form *and* technique. These functional movement parameters, key to your completion of the 12 Week Guide, are now with you – wherever you choose to go, and however and whatever movements you choose to perform. By being mindful of the functional movement parameters, your bodily control will be maintained whilst continually and consistently afforded natural strength and conditioning progressions with ease. There's no back-stepping here – it's your renewed lifestyle, and functional movement fitness is here to stay.

The freedom to create, make and choose – it's all yours. Your breakfast decisions – these are a continuous work in progress and afford you time to *think*: how does it make me *feel*, does it give me the *energy* I need, and, do I *like* it? Some days you would have answered "yes" to all three questions, other days there will be, and would have been a "no" – it's all a part of the learning process and you taking the responsibility, and the reins of your renewed lifestyle.

At the commencement of Part 4 it was a prerequisite for you to *define you reason*. By following the SMARTIE principle, you were able to ensure these goals were: *specific, measurable, achievable, realistic, time efficient, interesting*, and *enjoyable*. And herein hold the key then, now and going forward.

You now have *goals* that were ticked, whilst others are still on the list for you to achieve – and you will. By ensuring these goals, you *reason*, is *measurable* and *time efficient*, affords you a time-frame and performance indicator to accomplish your goal. This is *not* set in stone – it can be tweaked, but it is up to you, and being honest with *yourself* on how important this goal is to you, to achieve. This is where *achievable* and *realistic* come into play. Providing that your goals *are* something you believe in and that you believe you are capable of – nothing is holding you back. By setting goals that are interesting and enjoyable ultimately hold the key – they ensure these goals are a want and that you have the drive to achieve them. Hence, all in all, by following these principles, all of your goals are specific – they were and *are* your own personal road map, then, now and going forward.

Throughout your 12 Week Journey you were continuously asked questions – not by me, but by *you*! *Can I do it, can I keep going, is it all worth it, can I eat this, I really want to binge, maybe I'll just start again next week*, or *maybe this isn't for me*? This is just a handful of questions that more often than not you asked yourself – some of you perhaps some, or none – others all, plus a variety more; it doesn't matter. Some of you will have more bumps and bruises than others, some of you a little scruffy, others of you basking in the "blood, sweat and tears" – you are all different, we are all different, and regardless of "how" – you did, *you conquered*. You made – you made it through the 12 Weeks – you did, no one else, you finished what you started –that's all that counts. Be proud. Be proud of *you* and know that I am *incredibly* proud of you!

PART 5

YOUR LIFE

Outline

You came, you saw, applied and implemented – and conquered. This 12 Week Journey is no mean feat, but alas – here you are! The next phase of your renewed lifestyle is well under way and now it is all about *securing* that transition and allowing the Guide herein to form the basis, the back-bone, the foundations of your lifestyle.

If you've managed to do it for the past 12 Weeks – that's all it takes, *plus* more, to form a preordained habit. You're already a step ahead. The tools you have acquired throughout the Guide, alongside the "experience" and its implementation – through breakfast *and* weekend meal freedom, you *are* equipped to go forward, *without* set a set nutrition or fitness Guide. But, let the Guide *be used* at your discretion – it is at your disposal to use, tweak and modify for your lifestyle.

Going forward, when it comes to your nutrition you now have a gut *on* track – commencing its restoration and rejuvenation. This means the job isn't quite done – restoring your gut health takes time, depending on the state of your initial health and some may take longer than others due to a variety of influential factors. Most significantly, your gut has taken extensive progressions to be on its way. Are you there yet? This is at your discretion – ask yourself how you feel, how do you feel when consuming certain energy sources in contrast to others? Yet, this is a reminder – it's all about lifestyle, no "been" and "gone".

As you introduce "more" foods back into your diet, you will notice that your body may no longer like these or respond the same as it once did. Equally, you will find your body is at its most *optimal* when practicing and implementing what it has become accustomed towards – fitness, consistently maintaining and improving your *optimal wellbeing*.

5.1 Sticking to it

The Guide formed the beginning of your renewed lifestyle – giving you the tools and the power to regain control over your health *and* fitness. Now, the reins have been passed to you. What you have learned through *freestyle nutrition* is now yours to run with – you know now what is "good" for your body and what your body doesn't necessarily like by how it responds and how it makes you feel, reacts. The parameters of functional movement fitness are also now ingrained – they have become near second nature, innate in time if not already, and the "30 minutes" strength and "30 minutes" aerobic is *specific, measurable, achievable, realistic, time efficient*, and it is in your hands to ensure these minutes are *interesting* and *enjoyable* – for you. You can stick to it – you *will* stick to it, if your *reason* is yours and *yours* alone.

Your level of empowerment will surge. To be empowered, you need to take control – but I'll be right here. AM8 International (am8international.com) has been designed to provide you with ongoing tools on a more *refined* scale. This means, if you're ever unsure, or want to brainstorm "how" you're going to achieve your set *goals* behind your *reason*, I'm here: to help you. Regardless of where you are based around the world, AM8 International has solutions for you when called for – you'll never be alone.

5.2 Planning for the Future

It all starts with a plan and you're the director – and producer. The Guide was given to you to follow, to implement and to *learn* from – to prepare you for the future ahead. It is now your time to design your *own* Guide. To start, your goals *form* your reason, and in turn act as your *catalyst* for what your Guide comprises of and how it is to be executed.

The Guide in Part 4 acts as your blueprint – all you need to do is ask yourself: *how would I like to personalise it, more? How am I going to go about achieving my goals?* And, *how am I going to design my Guide to allow me to keep the reins of my optimal wellbeing?* This is your starting point – all you need to do is use the provided blueprint and shape it towards your wants *and* needs. There are no set rules – your body is the director; how it feels and responds will give you your answers, all you need to do is *listen*.

Ask. The journey doesn't stop here – it has merely just begun! You now have in your hands the blueprint for your renewed lifestyle and "how" to keep it not only intact, but to choose to commit to the heathier and fitter you. But there *will be* questions. You'll question if you're doing this right, if you should be doing "this" over "that", or uncertainties may arise. When this time comes – trust in yourself. When that trust wavers, I'll personally be around to reinstall and reaffirm that trust – a click away: AM8 International (am8international.com) is my *home* base that I am welcoming you *into* – a *global* point of contact where *I am*, willing and wanting to *help* you maintain, and continuously achieve, your *optimal wellbeing*.

5.3 Happiness and Health

First and foremost, it's your choice: happiness *and* health go hand in hand. Our endorphins – the body's natural "feel good" response, produced when we are happy *or* during and/or after physical activity, feed into our ultimate *optimal wellbeing*. Over the course of the past 12 Weeks your body's chemical response has been altered.

By beginning the Guide, your body not only went on a journey to restore and rejuvenate your gut health and lead you towards your *optimal wellbeing*, it also took on board activities that increased your heartrate, in a good way. From working towards continually improving your *gut health* in a simplified and less restrictive way, the Guide is designed for the long-term – for your renewed lifestyle, *not* a fad. The fitness component of the Guide has also prepared you for the long-term. By participating in activities that increased your heartrate – this contributes to how your body responds. Your heartrate, when under exertion, will continue to progressively improve, allowing you to increase load and/or intensity consistently. It also allows your body to more efficiently "function" – by lowering your heartrate, a cause-effect induced by partaking in physical activities, you are more readily able to disperse oxygen around your body; thus, getting less "puffed" over time. The list is endless.

The end result of improved nutrition and a consistent fitness schedule is internal *and* external. You would have noticed, and will continue to notice, your external transformation into a healthier and fitter you, whilst internally your body has and is becoming not only more efficient, from your heartrate to your metabolism, but you've ignited a catalyst and it's *still* going. And your happiness – has only started. The cause-effect of your health and its continuous improvement contributes to your happiness – all you need to do is *choose*. By choosing health and putting your health as a priority, your body will be "happy" and the endorphins you're continuously creating will become your norm, if not already, and happiness – it's the end result. Health *and* happiness – hand-in-hand.

Closing thoughts

*N*othing worthwhile ever comes easy* is a familiar phrase known by many, yet applied by few. *The Secrets to Optimal Wellbeing* is a Guide and its blueprint is now *with* you – for life. The lessons you have learned, the knowledge you have acquired, and the challenges you have faced – weren't easy – you made a choice to apply it and grab the reins of your lifestyle, choosing happiness *and* health. Because, you can have the "best" of *both* worlds.

The Road Map set out in Part 1 prepared you for the journey ahead – putting you in the director's chair and handing *you* a map. From here, you were able to tease through a variety of recipes in Part 2: Freestyle Nutrition, with various nutritional constraints in order to *revive* your gut, "shake" things up, and get your metabolism back on your *team*.

Come Part 3: Functional Movement Fitness, it was all about your fitness and "how" to move to ensure the Guide was in fact a lifestyle renewed, and not a lifestyle without longevity. Learning how to move functionally allowed you to, and has prepared you for, living here on in, and being, a healthier *and* fitter you.

Then the challenge was all yours – Part 4: Your 12 Week Journey, detailed what was to come for the next 12 Weeks – and *you came, you saw, you conquered*! There were goals set, reasons reaffirmed, and it was all about *you* – your choices, your freedom, you taking the reins, and you taking control *back* of your lifestyle and that lifestyle you choose – *towards a healthier and fitter you.*

And then you were here – Part 5: Your life, sticking to the lifestyle you *want*, and continuously working towards achieving it. Through planning, utilising the Guide herein as your blueprint, health and happiness are your *rewards* – your freedom to *choose*, your freedom to *control*, and your freedom to choose *happiness* – it's all yours.

Your future is now. May this Guide continue to restore and rejuvenate your gut – like it has mine; may it continuously push you towards a healthier and fitter you – like I continue to reap; and may it lead you towards a healthier *and* fitter you – like it did for me.

The Secrets to Optimal Wellbeing was written as a result of my health being taken away from me – whilst not one-person adept to give me answers on how to take control, again. I had to find these answers and *chose* to take back control. My guiding light? Happiness. No one deserves to be unhappy, no one deserves "not" to know – these don't have to be *secrets* no more. May *The Secrets to Optimal Wellbeing* continuously guide you and give you that elusive control you've been searching for – and may you always *choose* happiness.

Dr. B

WHAT NOW?

Visit https://AM8International.com and https://Topicthread.com for what's happening now and the latest resources available.

Want to get in touch? You can find Dr. B on Topicthread @Dr.B where she shares the latest news from Topicthread as well as her current running endeavours, publications, and performances.

BOOKS BY DR. B

The Secrets to Optimal Performance Success
(March, 2016)

The Secrets to Optimal Wellbeing
(September, 2016)

The Science of Elite Performance
(March, 2017)

The Secrets to Optimal Coaching Success
(March, 2018)

The Elite Research Method
(October, 2018)

What is Your Game Missing?
(March, 2019)

What is Your Game Missing, Now?
(October, 2019)

What is Your Game Missing, to Win?
(July, 2020)

I am Your Tennis Coaching Guru
(December, 2020)

The 7 Keys to Optimise Your Life
(December, 2021)

REFERENCE

AM8 International

The sporting world's leading developer of coach and athlete performance, providing resources and platforms for coach and athlete success, developing the best coaches and athletes in the world through publications and their partnership with Topicthread.

www.AM8International.com

www.ingramcontent.com/pod-product-compliance
Lightning Source LLC
Chambersburg PA
CBHW070241290326
41929CB00046B/2300